Migraine

Andrew J Dowson MB, BS
Director of the King's Headache Service,
King's College Hospital, London, UK

Roger K Cady MD
Director of the Headache Care Center &
Primary Care Network,
Springfield, Missouri, USA

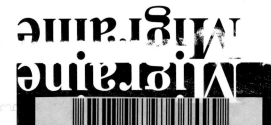

MOSBY

An affiliate of Elsevier Science Limited

ISBN 0-7234-3277-5

Cataloguing in Publication Data
Catalogue records for this book are available from the US Library of Congress and the British Library.

Note

Medical knowledge is constantly changing. As new information becomes available, changes in treatment, procedures, equipment and the use of drugs become necessary. The authors and publishers have, as far as it is possible, taken care to ensure that the information given in this text is accurate and up to date. However, readers are strongly advised to confirm that the information, especially with regard to drug usage, complies with latest legislation and standards of practice.

your source for books, journals and multimedia in the health sciences

www.elsevierhealth.com

The publisher's policy is to use paper manufactured from sustainable forests

Printed by Grafos S.A. Arte sobre papel, Spain

Acknowledgement

The authors wish to thank Dr Pete Blakeborough of Alpha-Plus Medical Communications Ltd for his help in the preparation of this book.

Contents

Introduction and Background

Introduction to headache in primary care

Managing patients with headaches in the primary care setting can, at times, be a daunting task. There is a widespread belief that it is a trivial condition. Patients rarely consult their doctor just for headache, either not consulting at all or mentioning it in passing at the end of a consultation for another condition. The doctor is often given little medical education on headache and is presented with what can seem to be a bewildering variety of conditions to diagnose and manage. Justifiably, they are most concerned with the exclusion or treatment of sinister, secondary headaches that may be life-threatening to the patient. However, most headaches encountered in primary care are straightforward to diagnose and manage. With a little education, many of the necessary management skills can be conducted by a practice nurse or pharmacist.

Headache is a very common condition. Almost all (96%) of the population suffer from headache at some time in their lives and approximately 70% have headache on at least a monthly basis. The vast majority of these disorders are primary headaches that resolve spontaneously without treatment, but which nevertheless can significantly limit the lifestyle of the sufferer. These headaches can be acute (intermittent) or chronic (continuous) in nature. The proportion of people who have sinister, secondary headaches is incredibly small. Headaches most frequently encountered in primary care include migraine, tension-type headache, short, sharp headache, cluster headache, chronic daily headache and sinus headache and other causes of facial pain.

Headaches frequently seen in primary care

Migraine is a common acute, intermittent headache that tends to be disruptive, with sufferers experiencing a significant loss in quality of life and an inability to perform their normal daily activities. Migraine affects at least 10% of adults, and is more common in women than in men.

Tension-type headache (TTH) is a very common acute, intermittent headache, but is generally not disabling and is relatively easily managed. About 50% of the population may be affected by these headaches on a monthly basis.

Short, sharp headache is an acute, intermittent headache that is much less common than migraine and tension-type headache, and often triggered by cold. For this reason, they are often called "ice cream" or "ice pick" headaches.

Cluster headache is a rare condition that can be acute or chronic in nature, and mostly affects men. It is characterized by relatively short-lived (15 minutes to 3 hours), but intensely painful headaches that occur several times a day for periods of weeks, months or on a daily basis. This condition is only present in about 0.25% of people.

Chronic daily headache (CDH), as the name suggests, comprises daily or near-daily headache that lasts for more than 4 hours and is often linked to analgesic overuse. It is relatively common, affecting about 5% of the population, and usually arise from a primary, acute headache disorder.

Facial pain: sinusitis headache is caused by infection of the cranial sinuses. It is relatively uncommon. However, it is often confused with migraine and tension-type headache. Other types of facial pain include *trigeminal neuralgia* (short, paroxysmal facial pain usually seen in the elderly), *post-herpetic neuralgia* after an eruption of herpes zoster and *temporomandibular joint dysfunction*.

Migraine

Migraine is the most frequently seen disabling headache in primary care. Until recently, relatively little was known about its causes, prevalence, distribution in society and impact on sufferers and the nation's economy. There have perhaps been more incorrect "myths" concerning migraine than any other medical condition. However, in the past dozen years, there has been an explosion of new information concerning the condition, and we now know what causes migraine, its natural history, who is affected and the extent of their suffering. This has coincided with the development and marketing of new, effective migraine therapies that have transformed migraine treatment.

This short book aims to provide the information necessary for the primary care doctor to manage migraine (and other common headaches) effectively. Firstly, we cover the current state of knowledge on the illness, its epidemiology, natural history, illness burden and underlying causes. We then move on to describe how to diagnose migraine and differentiate it from other common and uncommon headache disorders. Current practices of managing migraine are outlined and their pitfalls described, and an evidence-based guide as to the available choices of treatment for headache is provided. Synthesizing material from these two chapters, we then provide a practical guide for the overall management of migraine and other headaches in the primary care setting. Finally, we answer the questions most frequently asked by both doctors and patients and take a look at the future of headache research and clinical practice. The book is designed to be also used by practice nurses and pharmacists, who form an integral part of the primary healthcare team for headache.

Definition, Epidemiology and Natural History

Migraine is defined as a common, painful condition of recurring headache attacks, commonly accompanied by non-headache-associated symptoms.[1] Attacks are sometimes preceded by aura symptoms. Attacks are classified as *migraine with aura* and *migraine without aura*, depending on the presence or absence of these symptoms. The migraine headache lasts between 4 and 72 hours, with total freedom from symptoms between attacks. However, migraine is a heterogeneous disorder and attacks vary in their frequency, duration, severity and number of associated symptoms.

Epidemiology of migraine

Migraine is a common disorder, mostly affecting young and middle-aged people, and is more common in women than in men. Studies conducted around the world have consistently shown that migraine affects about 10–12% of the general adult population.[2] Migraine without aura is much more common than migraine with aura, accounting for about 90% of patients.[2] Migraine attacks usually start in childhood or adolescence; it is rare for new cases to occur at over 30 years of age. Migraine is two to three times more common in women than in men, presumed in part to be due to the influence of female hormones. However, peak prevalence occurs between the ages of 25 and 55 years for both genders (Figure 1).[3] Migraine is common in all races, but is more prevalent in white than in black or Asian races.[2] Results from the USA indicate that migraine prevalence is inversely associated with the level of education and social class.[3] However, this association was not observed in European and Canadian studies,[2] and therefore remains unproven.

Although migraine is a self-limiting illness and resolves without sequelae, it leads to significant morbidity by itself and in combination with associated conditions. Migraine is linked to certain psychiatric disorders (particularly major depression,

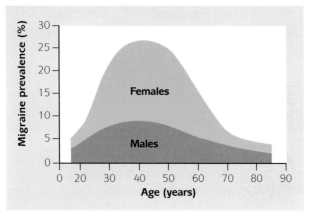

Figure 1. Prevalence of migraine. Reprinted from Staffa JA, Lipton RB, Stewart WF. *Rev Contemp Pharmacother* 1994; **5**: 241–252 with permission from the Marius Press.[26]

general anxiety, bipolar disorder and social phobia), epilepsy, stroke in women aged under 45 years and asthma.[2] Sufferers therefore experience the burden of associated illnesses as well as the migraine itself.

The natural history of migraine

The migraine attack involves a cascade of neurological, psychological and physical changes that generally occur in a predictable manner. Clinically, the acute attack is divided into five phases that occur in series: *prodrome*, *aura*, *headache*, *resolution* and *recovery* (Figure 2).[4]

Prodrome

This pre-headache phase is characterized by non-specific symptoms such as:
- Tiredness and yawning.
- Mood disruption.
- Muscle pain.
- Food cravings.
- Heightened perception.
- Fluid retention.
- Cognitive disruption.

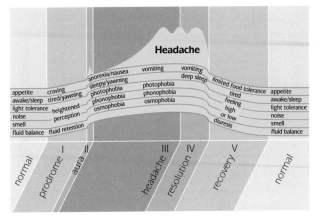

Figure 2. The five phases of the migraine attack: prodrome, aura, headache, resolution and recovery (adapted from reference 4).

Prodrome symptoms occur before about 50–70% of migraine attacks and last for several hours to several days. Patients may not be aware of the significance of these symptoms unless educated about them. However, the majority of migraine sufferers can predict at least some of their migraine attacks by these symptoms.[5] Some of the symptoms, e.g. muscle tension, food cravings and heightened sensory awareness, may be mistaken for migraine *triggers* (see pp. 28–29) by the patient. Prodrome symptoms arise presumably due to neurochemical disruption. They often continue throughout the attack, but are overshadowed by the headache phase.

Aura
Only about 10% of migraine sufferers experience aura symptoms, and not in all their attacks. Aura symptoms are reversible, localized neurological symptoms that are variable in timing and symptomatology. These symptoms typically last up to 1 hour, usually immediately precede the onset of headache, and may include:
- Visual disturbances (temporary blind spots, blurred vision, scotomas or a pattern of flashing lights or zigzag lines)(Figure 3).

Blurred, cloudy vision	Zigzag lines
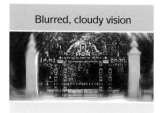	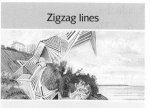

Figure 3. Typical visual aura symptoms reported by patients.

- Speech disturbances such as word-salading.
- Sensations affecting other areas of the body, such as tingling, dizziness, numbness, sensory loss and limb weakness.[4,6]

However, aura symptoms can also occur on their own without headache sequelae, can overlap with the prodrome and

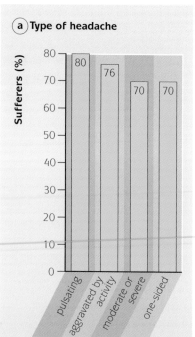

Figure 4. Headache- and non-headache-associated symptoms of the headache phase of the migraine attack (adapted from reference 7).

headache, or there can be a gap between the prodrome and aura.[4,6] The presence of aura symptoms is not predictive of the severity of the following headache. Attacks of migraine without aura may be as, or more, severe than those of migraine with aura. Auras are believed to occur due to electrical events initiated by a wave of spreading cortical depression.

Headache

The headache phase of migraine is characterized by headache that usually starts with mild (dull, diffuse) pain, but which can escalate to moderate or severe disabling pain that leads to disruption of the sufferer's normal activities. The following symptoms are typically reported (Figure 4):

- *Headache* – the most prominent feature, which is usually throbbing, unilateral, aggravated by activity and moderate to very severe in intensity.

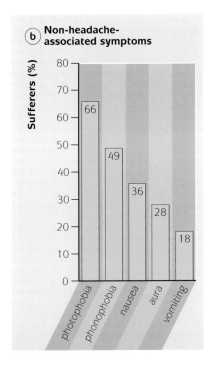

- *Photophobia and phonophobia* – reported by the majority of sufferers, which may cause them to have to lie down in a darkened room until the attack ends.
- *Nausea* – reported by half or more of sufferers.
- *Vomiting* – reported by 20% or less of sufferers, but indicative of a particularly severe attack.[7]
- Other symptoms suggesting autonomic activation are also seen, such as nasal congestion, rhinorrhoea, lacrimation and diarrhoea.

Both the frequency and duration of migraine attacks are highly variable. The average frequency is about one to two attacks per month, but may vary from <1 to >50 attacks per year (Figure 5).[3] The average duration is about 24 hours, but varies from <4 hours to several days (Figure 6).[1]

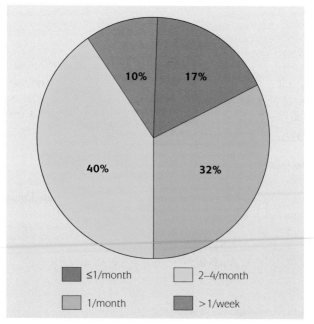

Figure 5. Average frequency of migraine attacks (data abstracted from reference 8).

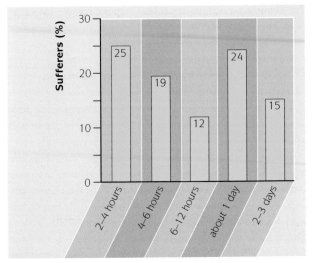

Figure 6. Average duration of migraine attacks (data abstracted from reference 8).

Resolution

After the headache peaks in intensity, it may gradually lessen and disappear over a period of hours. Sometimes, however, resolution may be triggered by a bout of vomiting, or sufferers may settle into a period of deep sleep and wake up with the symptoms gone.

Recovery

This final post-headache phase is characterized by lingering symptoms, much like a hangover without the headache. These include:

- Gastrointestinal symptoms with a sick, queasy stomach and food intolerance.
- Decreased concentration and occasional cognitive difficulties.
- Sore muscles.
- Overall sense of fatigue.

These symptoms can lead to disruption to the sufferer's normal activities, similar to a hangover (they are often called the "migraine hangover"). In contrast, some sufferers experience euphoria and a sense of well-being. The recovery phase can last from several hours to 48 hours.[5]

Burden of disease due to migraine

Migraine is a heterogeneous disorder characterized by attacks that vary in frequency, duration, severity and symptomatology. This variability exists both between different sufferers and within the individual sufferer over their separate attacks.[8] Migraine sufferers experience disability and reduced quality of life (QOL) during their attacks, which, over a lifetime's illness, can lead to profound consequences on their lifestyles.

Migraine-related disability

Migraine is a remarkably disabling condition, with most sufferers reporting significant impact associated with their attacks in all areas of their lifestyles. Migraine-related disability can be considered as the objective effects of the illness on sufferers' lifestyles, including their work and leisure activities, rather than subjective effects expressed as symptoms and QOL. Disability is defined by the World Health Organization as "a restriction or lack (resulting from an impairment) of ability to perform an activity in the manner or within the range considered normal for a human being".[9] Studies from around the world have shown that migraine causes significant disability in its sufferers, with two-thirds or more reporting at least mild disability and one-third or more reporting moderate to severe disability (Figure 7).[8] In a UK study, two-thirds of migraine sufferers reported that migraine disrupted their lives, with three-quarters having to lie down during attacks (Table 1).[10] A second study indicated that between one-third and two-thirds of migraine sufferers in the UK (an estimated 1.9–3.8 million people) felt that they were not in control of their migraine and the way it affected their day-to-day lives.[11]

The consequences of migraine-related disability are seen in patients' lifestyles, including employment, unpaid work, and family and leisure activities. The loss of these activities has been quantified in a series of studies. In the USA, each working

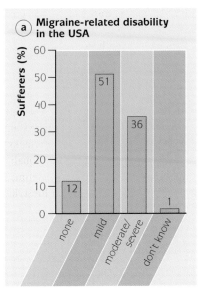

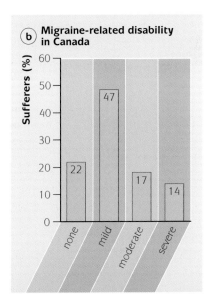

Figure 7. Migraine-related disability reported in studies conducted in the USA (a),[8] Canada (b)[39] and Japan (c)[42] (data abstracted from references 8, 39 and 42).

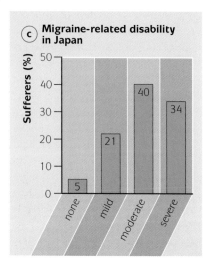

Impact of migraine on sufferers' lifestyles in the United Kingdom[10]	
Disability	**Proportion of sufferers (%)**
Physical functioning	
Always have to lie down	76
Not in control of life	34
Disruption of life	67
Employment	
Usually miss work	50
Difficulty performing work	72
Cancel appointments/meetings	67
Rely on other people	45
Perceived effect on promotion	15
Unpaid work	
Postpone household chores	90
Family and leisure activities	
Relations with family and friends affected	54

Table 1. Impact of migraine on sufferers' lifestyles in the United Kingdom.[10]

migraine sufferer missed an average of 4.4 days of work per year and the equivalent of 12 further days due to reduced productivity during attacks.[12] In the UK, half of sufferers reported missing work and over two-thirds reported difficulty performing work during attacks (Table 1).[10] Migraine may even lead to unemployment. In a primary care organization in the USA, the unemployment rate was two- to four-fold higher in severely affected migraine sufferers than in the general population (Figure 8).[13] School and college work is also affected in young migraine sufferers. In a Scottish study, children with migraine were absent from school for significantly longer periods than those without migraine (7.8 days versus 3.7 days per year, $p<0.0001$).[14] This personal burden of migraine is reflected in an economic burden on society. Indirect costs (due to work absence and reduced work productivity) are very large for migraine, being estimated as equivalent to about $0.5–13 billion per year in large Western countries (Table 2).[15] These costs are much higher than the direct costs due to medical care, estimated at about $15 million to $1 billion (Table 3).[15] Although direct medical costs for migraine have increased recently, partly due to the introduction of new drugs, indirect costs still provide the main economic burden of the illness.

Migraine also affects unpaid work and family and leisure activities. In a UK study, 90% of migraine sufferers reported that they postponed their household work during an attack (Table 1).[10] Several studies have shown that migraine attacks commonly result in the cancellation of social events, and affect relationships with partners, children, friends and other people.[10,16,17]

Effects on QOL

The QOL of migraine sufferers during their attacks is significantly poorer than that of the general healthy population, especially with respect to pain and interference to their daily and social lives (Figure 9).[18] In certain respects, it is also poorer than QOL in other chronic diseases that are usually considered to be more serious than migraine, such as hypertension, depression, osteoarthritis and type 2 diabetes (Figure 10).[18]

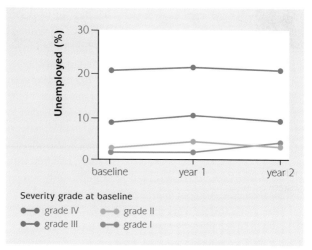

Figure 8. Association of migraine with unemployment in the USA (data abstracted from reference 13).

Indirect medical costs associated with migraine in Western countries[15]

Total annual indirect costs of migraine due to lost productivity (adjusted to US$)

USA	= $13 billion
Sweden	= $1.6 billion
UK	= $1.1–1.3 billion
Netherlands	= $1.2 billion
Spain	= $1.1 billion
Australia	= $568 million

Table 2. Indirect medical costs associated with migraine in Western countries.[15]

Direct medical costs associated with migraine in Western countries[15]	
Total annual costs of medical care (adjusted to US$)	
USA	= $1 billion
Sweden	= $13 million
UK	= $45 million
Netherlands	= $300 million
Australia	= $31 million

Table 3. Direct medical costs associated with migraine in Western countries.[15]

Moreover, migraine sufferers experience sub-optimal QOL even when they are symptom-free between attacks.[19]

Disease consequences of migraine

Anxiety, depression and fear are common among migraine sufferers, either as a direct result of the condition or due to coexisting psychiatric disorders.[2,20] In the long term, feelings of guilt, helplessness and despair can occur when sufferers see no end to the illness or think no effective treatment is available. There are many anecdotal accounts from sufferers of people losing their jobs and being divorced as a direct result of their migraine.[21]

The causes of migraine

The underlying causes of migraine have only recently been elucidated, and are still not completely understood. *Genetic*, *vascular* and *neural* components are all involved. Certain biochemical and physiological *risk factors* are hypothesized to predispose sufferers to migraine. Finally, many precipitating (*trigger or risk*) factors are proposed to initiate specific attacks. Figure 11 illustrates the interactions between these causative factors.

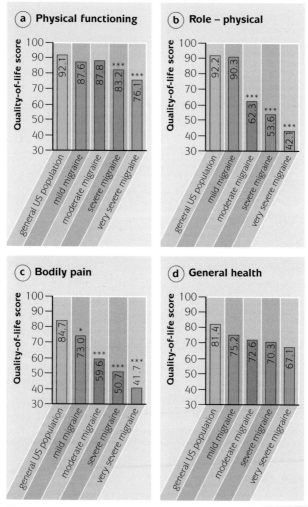

Figure 9. Quality of life of migraine sufferers compared with the general healthy population, *p≤ 0.05; ***p≤ 0.001 (data abstracted from reference 18).

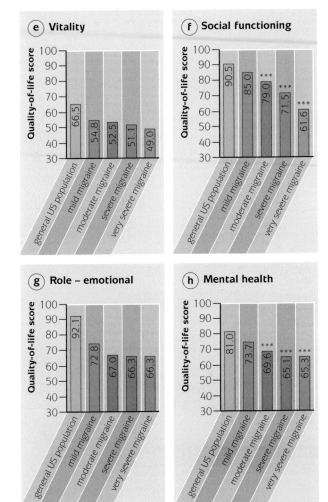

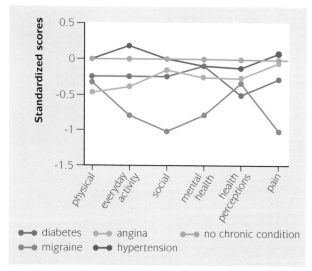

Figure 10. Quality of life of migraine sufferers compared with other chronic diseases (data abstracted from reference 18).

Genetic factors

Migraine has long been observed to "run in families", which gave impetus to investigations into the genetic nature of the disease. However, inheritance of migraine is complex. Migraine with aura seems to be determined by genetic factors whilst migraine without aura is determined by a combination of genetic and environmental factors.[22] Inheritance of migraine is multifactorial through several genes. Recent evidence has implicated a mutation in the gene for the voltage-dependent calcium ion channel protein on Chromosome 19 in migraine, as well as in other episodic and chronic neurological disorders. This indicates that migraine may be a form of channelopathy.[23]

The neurovascular theory of migraine pathogenesis

Two separate hypotheses have been proposed for explaining the pathogenesis of migraine: the vascular and the neural theories.

- The *vascular* theory proposes that migraine is caused by abnormal dilatation of cerebral vessels, possibly caused

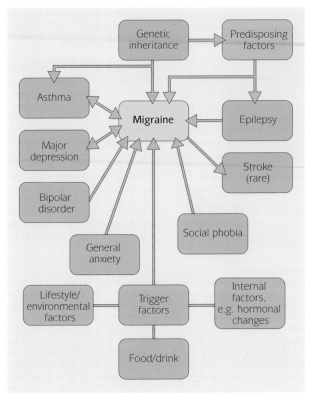

Figure 11. Overview of the relationship between migraine and genetic, predisposing and precipitating factors, and co-morbid illnesses (adapted from reference 2).

by decreased concentrations of blood 5-hydroxytryptamine (5-HT).

- The *neural* theory proposes that inflammatory mechanisms in the brain stem are responsible for initiating a migraine attack.

These two theories have now been combined into the *neurovascular hypothesis*, which incorporates components from both theories, and in which 5-HT plays a major role (Figure 12).[24]

When a susceptible nervous system confronts a migraine-provoking environment, neurochemical changes occur, often resulting in premonitory symptoms. Eventually, a critical threshold is reached and an area in the brain stem is activated (the hypothesized "migraine generator"; Figure 13).[25]

Increases in regional cerebral blood flow result, slightly opposite to the headache side.[24]

This stimulates sympathetic neurons and brain stem 5-HT- and noradrenaline-containing neurons to induce dilatation in intracranial blood vessels such as those in the meninges and large cerebral arteries.

These arteries are pain sensitive via a large innervation through sensory nerves in the trigeminal ganglion.

Activation of these sensory nerves causes the release of the inflammatory mediators substance P and calcitonin gene-related

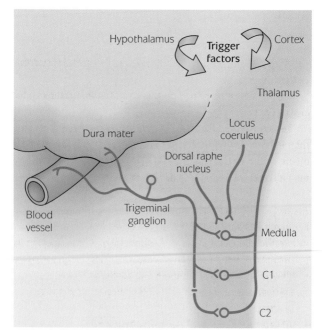

Figure 12. The neurovascular theory of migraine pathogenesis (adapted from reference 24).

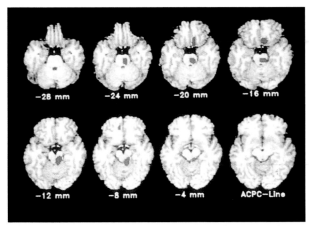

Figure 13. Possible site of the "migraine generator" in the brain stem. Reprinted from Weiller C, May A, Limmroth V et al. *Nature Med* 1995; **1**: 658–660, with permission from the Nature Publishing group.[25]

peptide (CGRP), which produce inflammation and distension of the vessel.

These stimuli produce pain signals that are transmitted centrally via the trigeminal nerve.

The nausea and/or vomiting commonly associated with migraine may be triggered by 5-HT release within the vomiting centre of the brain. These and other non-headache symptoms may also be caused by autonomic activation.

Predisposing risk factors

Research has shown that migraine sufferers can have certain metabolic abnormalities that have been hypothesized to predispose them to migraine. These identified factors include:

- Changes to platelet structure and function.
- Dysfunction and instability in the autonomic nervous system.
- Abnormal function of the opiate receptor.
- Changes in ovarian hormone levels.
- Decreased enzyme activities.[26]

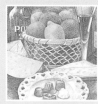

Food and drink
e.g. chocolate, cheese,
alcohol (especially red
wine), citrus fruits

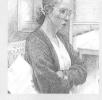

Stress
anxiety, tension, excitement,
depression, shock and frustration
may all lead to migraine attacks

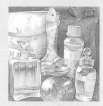

Strong smells
e.g. perfume, petrol, paint

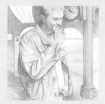

Irregular meals

Environmental factors
changes in the weather and
excessive heat, light or noise
may precipitate an attack

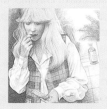

Hormonal changes
migraine may be associated
with the use of oral
contraceptives, menstruation,
puberty, the menopause or
pregnancy

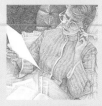

Sleep
too little or too
much sleep can
precipitate
migraine

Figure 14. Common migraine trigger factors. Reprinted with
permission from reference 32; copyright MIPCA, 1998)

However, the relevance of these abnormalities to migraine pathogenesis is not clear. Without further evidence, the coexistence of migraine and these putative risk factors may be purely coincidental.

Migraine trigger factors

Most migraine attacks occur spontaneously. However, some internal and/or external stimuli are implicated in the precipitation of certain attacks. These are known as *trigger or risk factors*. Common migraine triggers are illustrated in Figure 14, and include foodstuffs, stress, smells, lifestyle and environmental factors, and hormonal changes.[27]

While trigger factors certainly play a role in the genesis of some patients' attacks, there is often little objective evidence to substantiate their general prevalence. For example, there are no good quality studies to substantiate the belief that foodstuffs can induce migraine attacks. An alternative explanation is that in the *prodrome* phase of the migraine attack, sufferers sometimes have cravings for certain foods or drinks (see pp. 10–11).[5] These may then be blamed for causing the attacks, when they are in fact a consequence of them.

Migraine and chronic daily headache

Migraine can be confused with chronic daily headache (CDH) in clinical practice. Patients experiencing very frequent headaches (present on >15 days of each month) that last for more than 4 hours are unlikely to have migraine alone, but probably have chronic daily headache.[1] Chronic daily headache is relatively common, affecting about 5% of the population.[28] The condition may arise as migraine or episodic tension-type headache, which subsequently becomes altered in character due to:

- Overuse of analgesics or ergotamine preparations taken for a primary headache disorder.[29] There is the potential for the development of a "spiral" of increasing headache frequency, analgesic overuse, development of rebound headaches and eventually chronic headache.
- As a result of head or neck injury occurring at any time in the sufferer's lifetime.[30]

The typical clinical picture is one of episodic migraine symptoms superimposed on a background of tension-type headache symptoms (Figure 15). The diagnosis and management of chronic daily headache are also different from those of migraine, and are discussed later in this book.

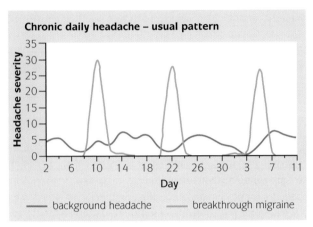

Figure 15. Typical profile of chronic daily headache over time. Reprinted with permission from reference 32; copyright MIPCA, 1998).

Diagnosis

The first step in the effective management of headache is to make the correct diagnosis when the patient first consults. It is important that the patient is made to appreciate that they have a recognized disorder that is not trivial and which the primary care physician appreciates is distressing. Fortunately, recent diagnostic advances mean that the physician has clear guidelines for the differential diagnosis of migraine and other headaches.

Migraine diagnosis

The International Headache Society (IHS) published definitive diagnostic guidelines for migraine and other headache types in 1988.[1] These guidelines have transformed research into migraine and the management of the condition by providing a standardized means of identifying migraine patients for physicians. According to these criteria, migraine is a diagnosis of both inclusion and exclusion: inclusion because certain features must be present, and exclusion because secondary headaches must be eliminated as a prelude to diagnosis. The IHS recommendations for migraine diagnosis are shown in Table 4.

From the above, it is important to note that no single headache feature and no single non-headache symptom are absolutely required for diagnosis. For example, a patient with severe bilateral headache associated with photophobia and phonophobia can be diagnosed with migraine, just as the more typical patient with unilateral headache accompanied with nausea. Migraine diagnosis using the IHS criteria is therefore somewhat of an art and requires a flexible approach rather than the simple "ticking of boxes".

Diagnosis of aura

For a migraine attack to be classified as migraine with aura, the IHS defines the following additional diagnostic criteria for the diagnosis of aura symptoms:

The International Headache Society criteria for the diagnosis of migraine[1]
The occurrence of five or more lifetime headache attacks with similar features lasting from 4 to 72 hours each, patients being symptom-free between attacks (these criteria help to exclude secondary headaches, which are less likely to recur without sequelae).
The presence of two or more of the following headache features: • Moderate to severe pain. • Pain on one side of the head. • Throbbing or pulsating headaches. • Headaches exacerbated by routine activities (such as climbing stairs).
The presence of one or more non-headache-associated symptoms: • Aura symptoms. • Nausea during the headache. • Photophobia and/or phonophobia during the headache.
The exclusion of secondary headaches, by a search for "headache alarms", by history taking or physical examination (see pp. 34–37).

Table 4. The International Headache Society criteria for the diagnosis of migraine.[1]

- The presence of at least three of the following four characteristics:
  - one or more fully reversible aura symptoms (see pp. 11–13);
  - one or more aura symptoms develop gradually over more than 4 minutes, or two or more symptoms occur in succession;
  - no single aura symptom lasts more than 60 minutes;
  - the migraine headache occurs less than 60 minutes after the end of the aura symptoms.

In addition, secondary (sinister) headaches have to be excluded as the cause of the aura symptoms.[1]

Migraine diagnosis in primary care

The IHS diagnostic guidelines were developed by a group of neurologists and headache specialists as a definitive means of diagnosing migraine and other headaches. They are now widely used by researchers for studies on migraine around the world and clinically in specialist neurology and headache clinics. Used appropriately, the IHS guidelines can be used to diagnose migraine definitively and differentiate it from other headache disorders.

However, full application of the IHS diagnostic guidelines is a lengthy process. Primary care physicians, who have restrictions on the time they can give to each patient, will usually find them too cumbersome for routine use. Also, most headaches that primary care physicians encounter are due to the common disorders of migraine, tension-type headache and chronic daily headache. Other headaches are rare and will be seen only occasionally, if ever. The primary care physician needs:

- A means of identifying patients with rare or secondary (sinister) headache who are best referred to a specialist.
- A simple and rapid means of diagnosing migraine and other common headaches.

Although over 95% of the population experience headaches, a very small proportion of these headaches have sinister pathology. However, a critical aspect of diagnosing the symptoms of headache in the primary care setting is to separate primary headaches from headaches that are secondary to underlying disease. This is most efficiently accomplished by looking at the pattern of headaches a person presents with. In the medical setting a stable pattern (greater than 6-month history) of recurrent episodes of headaches that disrupt a person's function should be considered migraine until proven otherwise. The following data and observations support this statement:

Most significant sinister headaches are new in onset or differ from the established pattern of headache an individual experiences.

Low-impact headaches, unless chronic (not recurrent), do not reach a threshold where medical consultation is sought.[31]

People with migraine rarely have a stereotyped headache pattern, but almost inevitably experience a variety of headache presentations from migraine to migraine-like and tension-type headache. All of these different presentations are reflections of the migraine process and respond in a similar fashion to migraine-specific medications.

Making the initial diagnosis at the patient's first consultation is the first key step in the effective management of migraine. This can be accomplished simply and rapidly using the following scheme:

- Migraine headaches are generally acute, painful episodes of headache that significantly affect patients' QOL and their ability to perform normal activities.
- In contrast, tension-type headache tends to not impact significantly on the patient's lifestyle.
- Chronic daily headache, by definition, is a chronic (occurring on a daily or near-daily basis) rather than an acute disorder.

Any episodic, high-impact, acute headache can therefore be given an initial default diagnosis of migraine, and the IHS diagnostic criteria can then be used to confirm this. Rather than using the IHS criteria as published, the physician can ask the series of questions shown in Table 5. An affirmative answer to most questions confirms the diagnosis as migraine.[32]

Differential diagnosis of non-migraine headaches
Sinister headaches

Primary care physicians worry about misdiagnosing presenting headache symptoms as indicative of serious underlying pathology, although patients presenting with these conditions are rare. Patients, too, may be worried that their headache is caused by a brain tumour or other life-threatening disorder. However, the physician should realize that the majority of headache sufferers who seek advice have the common, high-impact headaches of migraine or chronic daily headache. Nevertheless, there are certain symptoms indicative of sinister headaches requiring referral that can be elicited straightforwardly by the primary care physician:

Key questions that can be used to diagnose migraine in primary care[32]
Headache characteristics
Does the headache last between 4 hours and 3 days?
Does the patient suffer from headache on more than 15 days each month?
Does the patient feel well between attacks?
Is the headache a throbbing, pulsating pain?
Is the headache located on one side of the head at any stage?
Non-headache-associated symptoms
Does the patient suffer from wavy lines, flashing lights or blind spots affecting their vision before or during the headaches?
Does the patient feel sick or vomit during their headaches?
Does the patient feel that they want to avoid light and/or noise during their headaches?
Headache impact
Does the patient desire to lie down when they have a headache?
Is the patient prevented from, or have difficulties in, conducting their normal daily activities (employment, unpaid work and leisure activities) when they have a headache?

Table 5. Key questions that can be used to diagnose migraine in primary care.[32]

- Age of the patient – those having their first or worst headache at the age of >50 years.
- Headache on wakening, especially in children.
- Persistent headache in children.
- Pain or tenderness over the temporal artery, especially in patients >50 years.
- A change in the patient's pattern of headaches.
- Symptoms or signs additional to the headache, especially if they occur between the patient's headaches, e.g. progressive neurological symptoms.

- An acute onset of headache, especially when associated with vomiting.
- Headache following an accident or head injury.
- Headache with a fever or stiff neck.
- Headaches (usually occipital) associated with uncontrolled hypertension.
- In general, sinister headaches, although constituting a vast minority of headaches reported, are generally new onset or different from the person's normal headaches.[33]

Some examples of sinister headaches and their diagnostic pointers are shown in Table 6.

Tension-type headache

Tension-type headache is often confused with migraine both by the patient and the physician. Key ways of distinguishing tension-type headache are as follows:

- The headache is typically bilateral, mild to moderate in intensity, and may persist for longer periods than migraine.
- The headache is low impact, patients being able to work and function fairly normally throughout the attacks.
- Associated symptoms: one, but not both, of photophobia or phonophobia may be present, but these are usually mild in intensity. There is no associated nausea or vomiting.[1]
- Episodic tension-type headache that produces disability is uncommon in medical practice.[31]

Short, sharp headache

Features of this headache subtype include:

- Patients are often young to middle-aged adults.
- The pain is piercing, very severe, short-lived, lasting from seconds to minutes (most commonly 15–30 seconds) and usually centred on one eye.
- Patients often feel slightly bruised after the pain has resolved.
- Patients can have multiple attacks during the day.
- The pain is frequently, but not always, triggered by eating ice cream or other cold foods.[34]

Sinister headaches: diagnostic pointers	
Possible diagnosis	**Sinister headache pointing to diagnosis**
Meningitis	• First presentation • Acute headache with rash
Subarachnoid haemorrhage	• First presentation • Acute headache with vomiting and photophobia
Cranial arteritis	• First presentation • Headache associated with jaw pain, scalp and muscle tenderness, and general malaise • Occurs particularly in Caucasians aged >60 years and Afro-Caribbeans aged >50 years
Space-occupying lesions: primary brain tumour	• Headache with symptoms or signs suggestive of ongoing neurological deficit between headache attacks
Space-occupying lesions: cerebral metastases	• Headache with neurological signs/deficit • History of malignancy
Space-occupying lesions: cerebral abscess	• Acute headache associated with neurological deficit, high or persistent fever and apparent infection of one or more systems

Table 6. Sinister headaches: diagnostic pointers.

Sometimes the headache lasts for over 3 minutes and diffusely affects one side of the head. This type of headache is termed chronic paroxysmal hemicrania.

Cluster headache

Cluster headache has similarities to migraine, but differs in the following characteristics:

The condition almost exclusively affects men.

- The pain is excruciating, unilateral and often concentrated around one eye. One or more autonomic features are always associated with the headache; the eyes may be red and watering, and there is often a blocked nose.
- Each attack lasts from 15 minutes to 3 hours, with an average of 45 minutes (i.e. shorter duration than migraine). Attacks have an abrupt onset and cessation.
- Attacks occur with a frequency ranging from once every other day to eight times daily, and often have a circadian rhythm.
- Most patients (80–90%) have attacks that usually occur in clusters over the course of 2–3 months separated by attack-free intervals lasting from months to years (episodic cluster headache).
- A minority of patients (10–20%) have symptoms for more than 1 year with pain-free periods of <14 days (chronic cluster headache).
- Alcohol rapidly induces cluster headaches in most sufferers.[35]

Chronic daily headache

Chronic daily headache has the following characteristic features:

- Very frequent headaches (>15 days per month) lasting more than 4 hours.
- Headaches present for 6 months or longer.
- Headaches are resistant to treatment.
- History of primary headache (migraine or tension-type headache) superimposed on a background of daily headache.
- Possible history of head or neck injury.
- Likely chronic overuse of headache medications such as analgesics or ergots.[28,29]

Facial pain

Acute sinusitis is a relatively uncommon cause of headache, but is greatly over-diagnosed due to confusion with migraine and tension-type headache. Key points allowing a correct diagnosis are:

- Purulent discharge from the nose.
- Evidence of acute febrile illness.
- Headache in the sinus areas occurring simultaneously with the sinusitis.
- Dull, aching headache exacerbated by bending down.
- Diminished smell (in migraine the sense of smell is usually heightened).[1]

Trigeminal neuralgia is the most common neurological syndrome in the elderly and is three times more common in women than in men. Characteristic diagnostic features include:

- Spasms of usually unilateral, intense, stabbing or burning pain along the trigeminal nerve lasting a few seconds to 2 minutes.
- Often provoked by activities such as washing, shaving, talking or brushing teeth.
- The patient is symptom-free between attacks.[1]

Post-herpetic neuralgia is characterized by the presence of pain after an eruption of herpes zoster. Symptoms include a constant, deep pain with repetitive stabs or needle-prick sensations, starting during the acute rash. Light touch can trigger the symptoms and lead to itching.[36]

Temporomandibular joint dysfunction can lead to pain in the upper part of the head, frequently migraine or tension-type headache.[36] Patients prone to jaw clenching or teeth grinding while asleep may be prone to this syndrome.

Current Migraine Management in Primary Care

Even though migraine is a significant personal and public health problem, it is not always managed effectively in primary care. This is largely due to variability of the condition on presentation.[8] A large proportion of migraine sufferers do not engage the healthcare system and, of those that do, many are given incorrect diagnoses and sub-optimal treatments (Figure 16). This section examines the reasons underlying this unsatisfactory situation,

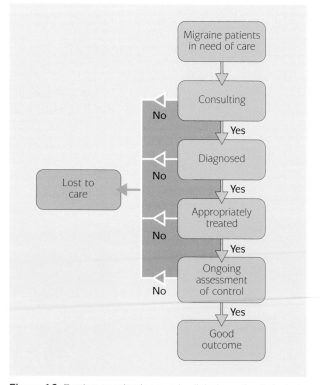

Figure 16. Barriers to migraine care in clinical practice (adapted from reference 164).

and proposes initiatives to improve strategies for managing migraine and other headaches in primary care.

Barriers to migraine care

Consultation patterns for migraine

The majority of migraine sufferers worldwide do not currently consult their physicians about the condition (Table 7).[7,38–42] A substantial proportion has never seen a physician about migraine. Nevertheless, many people who never consulted suffer significantly from their migraine. In one study, 60% of American women reported severe to very severe pain and 68% reported severe disability or were forced to rest in bed during

Consultation patterns for migraine: results from population-based epidemiological studies			
Study area	**Proportion of patients (%)**		
	Ever consulted	**Current consulter**	**Lapsed consulter**	**Never consulted**
UK, 1999[38]	86	49	37	14
Canada, 1993[39]	81	36	45	19
USA, 1998[40]	67	47	21	32
International,* 1993[7]	66	31	35	34
Denmark, 1992[41]	56	ND	ND	44
Japan, 1997[42]	31	15	16	69

*Study conducted in Belgium, Canada, Italy, Sweden and the UK.
ND = no data

Table 7. Consultation patterns for migraine: results from population-based epidemiological studies (adapted from reference 50).

their attacks.[40] Of sufferers who do consult a physician, the pattern seems to be an initial consultation period of about 1 year, followed by a lapse in care-seeking behaviour thereafter.[43]

The main reasons given by migraine sufferers for not consulting include:

- A belief that there is nothing the physician can do to help.
- Dissatisfaction with the care received from their physicians.[38,39]

Diagnosis of migraine

Studies conducted in primary care in the USA and France showed that over half of migraine sufferers who consulted for headache (55% in the USA[44] and 58% in France[45]) did not receive an accurate diagnosis from their physician. In the UK, only 2% of consulting patients in two general practices had received a diagnosis of migraine in the previous 5 years,[46] whereas the expected figure from the known migraine prevalence should have been about 10%.[3] Patients who tended not to be diagnosed were:

- Men.
- Those with migraine without aura.
- Those with depression as well as migraine.
- Those without significant headache-related disability.

Treatment of migraine

Although many effective treatments are now available for migraine, the sufferer who consults a physician and receives an accurate diagnosis may still not receive appropriate therapy. Most migraine sufferers in Europe and North America rely on over-the-counter (OTC) medications, relatively few taking prescription drugs (Table 8).[39,47,48]

Furthermore, many migraine sufferers do not report effective relief with their anti-migraine medications. In the USA, only 29% of migraine sufferers stated that they were satisfied with their usual acute treatments. Features that led to dissatisfaction included:

- A lack of overall relief.
- Delay in the onset of relief.
- Too many side-effects.[49]

Proportion of migraine sufferers using prescription and OTC medications			
Study area	**Sufferers (%)**		
	Prescription medications	**OTC medications**	**No medications**
International,** 1999[47]	45*	58*	11
Canada, 1993[39]	44*	91*	ND
USA, 1992[48]	37	59	4

*Some sufferers took both prescription and OTC medications.
**Study conducted in France, Germany, Italy, Sweden, the UK, Canada and the USA.
ND = no data.

Table 8. Proportion of migraine sufferers using prescription and OTC medications (adapted from reference 50).

Unmet treatment needs for migraine in primary care

Migraine sufferers differ in their management needs, largely due to the variation in severity of symptoms and their impact on the sufferer.[8] Although severely affected sufferers tend to receive more medical care than those less affected, a significant proportion of those with severe pain and disability remain undetected, undiagnosed and under-treated in clinical practice. Initiatives are needed to improve migraine care in several areas to provide a service focused on the individual patient's needs:

- Migraine sufferers should be encouraged to engage with the healthcare system, to consult their primary care provider and receive appropriate treatment.
- Currently consulting migraine patients need to be motivated to continue with their care.
- Physicians require simple but comprehensive guidelines to allow them to diagnose migraine differentially from other headaches.

- Physicians should be encouraged to provide prescription medications that have been proven to be effective.[50]

The primary healthcare provider for migraine

The majority of headache management takes place in the primary care setting. Over 90% of headache cases in the UK[46] and over 50% of migraine cases in Denmark, the Netherlands, Canada and the USA[50] are dealt with initially by primary care physicians. Only a minority of cases need referral to a specialist. Other healthcare providers used by migraine patients as their initial point of contact include:

- Specialists, used by a minority of patients almost solely in the USA and Canada, include neurologists, gynaecologists, obstetricians, ophthalmologists, and pain and headache specialists.
- Hospital emergency rooms, again used significantly only in North America by a minority of patients.
- Alternative practitioners, e.g. physiotherapists, homeopaths and acupuncturists, used by a significant minority of patients in the USA and Europe.[49]
- Pharmacists, used by most headache sufferers and solely relied on by about 15% of sufferers internationally.[47]

As primary care physicians are the medical service most commonly used by migraine sufferers, it makes sense to coordinate headache management services around them. Unfortunately, the education of primary care physicians about headache is usually limited to the exclusion of serious but rare secondary (sinister) headaches rather than the management of very common benign primary headaches. Primary care physicians also have severe limitations to the time they can give each patient. Simple, clear and unified guidelines are therefore needed to allow the primary care physician to deal with patients with headache. The goals should be to:

- Accurately diagnose and provide appropriate treatment for the majority of patients who can be managed in primary care.
- Rapidly identify and refer the minority of patients who need to be seen by a specialist.

Management guidelines for migraine

Management guidelines for migraine have been published in many countries, including the UK,[51] USA[52] and Germany.[53] These guidelines, while comprehensive, are perhaps better suited for specialist use than in primary care. They tend to emphasize a rigorous diagnostic procedure, followed by a stepped or staged approach to care. Patients are moved through a sequence of medications, starting with low-end therapies and moving through stronger therapies until they find an effective treatment or lapse from care (Figure 17).[51–53] A typical scheme is for the patient to be started on a simple analgesic, followed by an analgesic combination (e.g. aspirin plus metoclopramide) and finally a

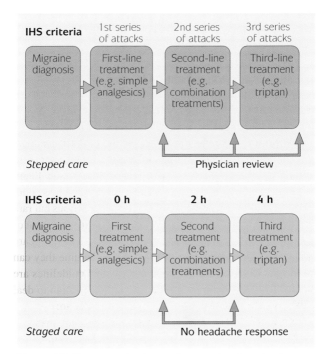

Figure 17. The stepped and staged approaches for migraine care (adapted from reference 56).

triptan. These guidelines require a significant investment in time and effort for the physician and the patient, with no guarantee of success in the short term. There is another, more subtle point, which can be described as "medicine is the art of the possible". After years of promotion of these guidelines, there have been no major inroads into the way many primary care physicians manage headache. The inescapable conclusion is that this recommended approach does not seem worthwhile to primary care physicians. There is a wide gap between what often happens in primary care practice and what specialists are recommending, the end result being the poor consultation, diagnostic and treatment success rates seen for migraine.

Recently, several initiatives have been undertaken to develop new guidelines for the management of migraine in primary care, including those issued by the Migraine in Primary Care Advisors (MIPCA) in the UK and the Headache Consortium and the Primary Care Network in the USA.

The Migraine in Primary Care Advisors (MIPCA) guidelines

The MIPCA guidelines were first issued in 1997, and then revised and published in 2000.[54] The MIPCA advocates an individualized approach to care, treatment being prescribed according to each patient's needs. Factors considered include the nature of the patient's attacks, the impact of headache on the individual's life and the demands of the patient's lifestyle (Figure 18).

At the initial consultation, the physician is recommended to conduct a diagnostic assessment and to take a careful history covering the nature of the headaches, previous treatments taken and the impact on the patient's life. Patients who experience up to four attacks per month are given acute therapy with a simple analgesic (with or without an anti-emetic) or an oral triptan if analgesics have been used unsuccessfully in the past. Nasal spray or subcutaneous triptan formulations may be considered if the patient has difficulties with oral therapies or requires a fast therapeutic effect due to the demands of their lifestyle or presentation characteristics of their headaches. It is essential to establish a goal for therapeutic intervention.

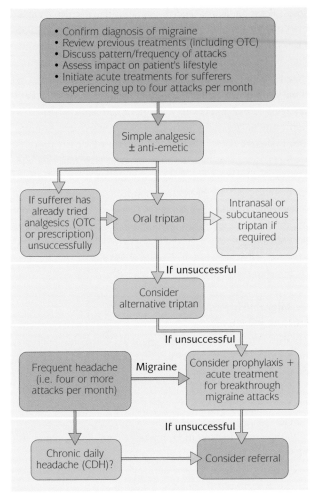

Figure 18. The MIPCA guidelines for migraine management. Reprinted with permission from reference 54; copyright MIPCA, 2000).

Useful goals centre on preservation of function or being free of pain and associated migraine symptoms. Merely providing enough relief to "get through" an attack commonly results in the patients lapsing from care.

If the initial therapy is unsuccessful, an alternative triptan may be provided. For patients who fail on this therapy, and for migraine patients with four or more headaches per month, prophylactic treatment is recommended with additional acute treatment for breakthrough attacks. Migraine patients who fail on this treatment, and those diagnosed with chronic daily headache, may require referral to a specialist physician.

The US Headache Consortium guidelines

New practice guidelines for the management of migraine were published by the US Headache Consortium in 2000.[55,56] Identified goals of successful migraine management were reduction of attack frequency, severity and disability, improvement of QOL, prevention of headache, avoidance of the escalation of acute medications and the education of patients to better self-manage their illness.

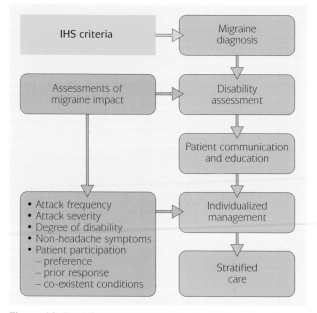

Figure 19. The US Headache Consortium guidelines for migraine management (adapted from reference 56).

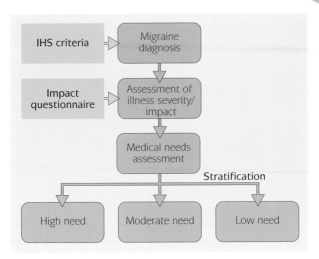

Figure 20. The stratified care approach for migraine care (adapted from reference 57).

The US Headache Consortium identified several principles for managing migraine (Figure 19).[55,56] Following a diagnostic assessment, the physician is recommended to assess the illness severity, by taking a history of attack frequency and severity, degree of disability, the presence of non-headache symptoms and patient-specific factors, such as their prior response to medications and coexistent conditions. A major part of these guidelines is the education of patients about their condition and its treatment, to establish realistic expectations and to encourage them to participate in the management of their migraine. Finally, an individualized treatment plan is advocated, tailoring therapy to the patient's symptoms, illness severity, disability and personal needs.

The US Headache Consortium mostly used evidence-based medicine to rate different treatments, but where this was not possible due to lack of data, a consensus was reached. They recommend a stratified approach to care, whereby the initial prescribed therapy is based on a baseline assessment of the illness severity and treatment needs of the patient (Figure 20).[57]

Non-steroidal anti-inflammatory drugs (NSAIDs) and combinations of analgesics with anti-emetics are recommended for patients with mild to moderate migraine. Migraine-specific agents (e.g. triptans) are recommended for patients with moderate to severe migraine and for those who have failed on NSAIDs and combination analgesics. The consortium advocates a non-oral route of administration for patients with severe nausea and vomiting and a rescue medication for treatment failures. Finally, physicians are cautioned to guard against the overuse of headache medications.

The US Primary Care Network guidelines

The Primary Care Network is a group of physicians working in private practice, managed care and academia, who provide medical programmes for the management of diseases in US primary care. They published a booklet on patient-centred strategies for managing migraine in 2000.[5] The Primary Care Network advocates the impact-based recognition of migraine and acute and preventative treatment strategies, together with special guidelines for using behavioural and physical treatments, treating chronic headache disorders and specific patient groups (Figure 21).

Impact-based recognition of migraine involves the physician eliciting information on how headaches interfere with the patient's life, the frequency of headaches, any changes in headache pattern over the preceding 6 months, and the previous use and effectiveness of headache medications (see pp. 119–121). The guidelines for acute treatment are to abort migraine symptoms and disability within 2–4 hours of initiating therapy. Key tactics for achieving this are identified as providing patient education and instruction and tailoring intervention to the individual's needs. The Primary Care Network recommends treating migraine early in the attack, when the headache is mild, with triptans, NSAIDs, isometheptene or combination analgesics. Migraine-specific treatments such as triptans are recommended if the headaches are likely to become moderate or severe (nearly 85% of patients with significant impact associated with their migraines have attacks that routinely

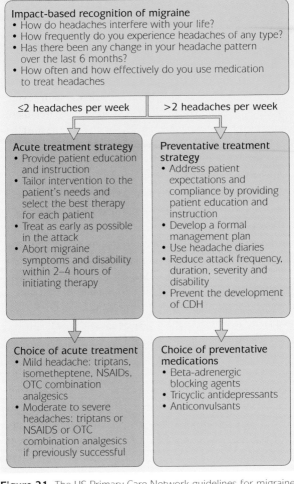

Impact-based recognition of migraine
- How do headaches interfere with your life?
- How frequently do you experience headaches of any type?
- Has there been any change in your headache pattern over the last 6 months?
- How often and how effectively do you use medication to treat headaches

≤2 headaches per week | >2 headaches per week

Acute treatment strategy
- Provide patient education and instruction
- Tailor intervention to the patient's needs and select the best therapy for each patient
- Treat as early as possible in the attack
- Abort migraine symptoms and disability within 2–4 hours of initiating therapy

Preventative treatment strategy
- Address patient expectations and compliance by providing patient education and instruction
- Develop a formal management plan
- Use headache diaries
- Reduce attack frequency, duration, severity and disability
- Prevent the development of CDH

Choice of acute treatment
- Mild headache: triptans, isometheptene, NSAIDs, OTC combination analgesics
- Moderate to severe headaches: triptans or NSAIDS or OTC combination analgesics if previously successful

Choice of preventative medications
- Beta-adrenergic blocking agents
- Tricyclic antidepressants
- Anticonvulsants

Figure 21. The US Primary Care Network guidelines for migraine management (adapted from reference 5).

become moderate to severe). This follows recent clinical trial evidence that early intervention with triptans when the migraine headache is mild is the most effective treatment option for migraine.[58] Preventative treatment is designed to reduce attack frequency, duration, severity and disability, and prevent the development of chronic daily headache in patients with frequent headaches. Again, this involves patient education and instruction, plus the development of a formal management plan.

These three sets of guidelines have several recommendations in common:

- Patient counselling should be provided and their buy-in sought.
- A careful diagnosis should be conducted.
- Assessments of migraine impact should be used in the initial evaluation of patients.
- An individual treatment plan should be produced for each patient.
- Patients who have disabling migraine are recommended to have access to migraine-specific therapies from the outset.
- Follow-up procedures should be implemented to monitor the outcome of therapy.

These general principles have application to all areas of headache management and will be used in the section on "Management of Migraine in the Primary Care Setting", where specific recommendations are made for the management of individual headache disorders.

Headache Treatments

Migraine therapies

Medications for the treatment of migraine can be given in two ways:

- Acutely for the symptomatic treatment of individual attacks.
- Prophylactically to prevent the development of future attacks.

"Alternative" therapies can also play a part, particularly for migraine prophylaxis. Lifestyle changes and behavioural therapies can be used as adjuncts to, e.g. reduce stress, alter the diet and change sleep patterns.

Acute medications are needed by all migraine sufferers for symptomatic treatment and, for the majority of patients who have infrequent attacks, are the only therapy required. Patients with frequent migraine attacks are usually also given a prophylactic medication. Although the definition of what constitutes "frequent migraine" requiring prophylaxis varies in different countries, patients with three or more attacks per month in the USA[59] or four or more attacks per month in the UK[53] are usually given migraine prophylaxis. However, as all prophylactic agents have limited efficacy and have the risk of chronic side-effects, an effective acute treatment is always required for the treatment of breakthrough attacks.

Medications can be prescribed or be available OTC without a prescription. The main classes of anti-migraine drugs are available in most countries, although individual medications can differ. Many anti-migraine medications have their efficacy and safety profiles proven in controlled clinical trials. However, evidence for the utility of some of the older medications and the "alternative" treatments tend to be much less robust.

Acute treatments for migraine

Commonly used acute treatments for migraine are listed in Table 9. Studies to evaluate acute treatments for migraine are now undertaken to unified and rigorous procedures to allow

Commonly used acute treatments for migraine	
Anti-emetics	Analgesic combinations

Analgesics
  Simple
  Opiate
	Ergots
	  Ergotamine
	  Dihydroergotamine

Barbiturates	Triptans

Table 9. Commonly used acute treatments for migraine.

the evaluation of results into treatment guidelines and the comparison of different medications. In brief:

- Studies are randomized, double-blind and placebo- or comparator-controlled.
- Patients are selected according to the IHS diagnostic criteria for migraine.[1]
- The primary end-point is headache relief, defined as a reduction from severe or moderate at baseline to mild or none at 2 hours after treatment.
- Other end-points include improvement in headache to pain-free, presence of nausea, vomiting and photophobia and phonophobia, improvement in the patient's functional abilities and the incidence of headache recurrence (where the headache is initially relieved at 2 hours, but subsequently deteriorates to severe or moderate over the 24-hour period after dosing).[60]

Anti-emetics
Anti-emetic drugs have been used for the acute treatment of migraine for some time as first-line therapy. However, clinical trials of monotherapy with oral domperidone, prochlorperazine and metoclopramide showed no clinical benefit.[55] Parenteral prochlorperazine and metoclopramide have demonstrated some efficacy, but are not usually used today as monotherapy for migraine. These drugs are well tolerated, with extrapyramidal side-effects (associated with the chronic use of metoclopramide) being reported rarely.

Analgesics

Simple analgesics

Simple analgesics such as paracetamol, aspirin and NSAIDs are usually the first treatment that patients try for migraine, as they are freely available without a prescription. Clinical trials have shown that aspirin and certain NSAIDs (ibuprofen, naproxen sodium and tolfenamic acid) have mild to moderate efficacy as acute treatments for migraine. However, there is no objective evidence of the efficacy of paracetamol in migraine.[55] Although these drugs are generally well tolerated, overuse can lead to analgesic rebound headache, and aspirin and NSAIDs can also cause gastrointestinal side-effects,[61] which can severely limit their use. The fact that these drugs can be used without any control from a physician is a potential public health issue and undoubtedly contributes towards the development of chronic daily headache.

Analgesic combinations

Simple analgesics are often combined with other medications in an attempt to improve their efficacy profiles for the acute treatment of migraine:

- *Caffeine* is added to attempt to improve the absorption of the analgesic.
- *Anti-emetics* such as domperidone and metoclopramide are added to prevent the gastric stasis often associated with migraine and to therefore improve the absorption of the analgesic. They may also reduce the nausea symptoms associated with migraine attacks.

Clinical trial data have shown that the following combination medications are moderately effective and well tolerated for mild to moderate migraine:

- Aspirin plus paracetamol plus caffeine (*not available in the UK*).
- Paracetamol plus domperidone (*not available in the USA*).
- Aspirin or paracetamol plus metoclopramide.[55]

Approximately 40–50% of migraine patients benefit from these combination drugs. In a controlled clinical trial, the combination of paracetamol plus domperidone was shown to have similar efficacy to oral sumatriptan (50 mg) in the treatment of moderate to severe migraine attacks.[62]

Opiate analgesics

The combination of codeine (16–25 mg) with paracetamol was shown to be effective for moderate to severe migraine in clinical trials.[55] However, adverse events included dizziness, drowsiness, fatigue and nausea. Codeine is also a major cause of analgesic rebound headache and chronic daily headache. Its use, therefore, needs to be limited to avoid the development of dependency.

Butorphanol nasal spray is used in some countries as a rescue medication for moderate to severe migraine when other treatments have failed. Clinical studies have demonstrated its efficacy in this role.[55] Adverse events are reported frequently and are similar to those described for codeine above. Again, frequent use can lead to analgesic rebound headache and chronic daily headache. (*Butorphanol is not available for migraine in the UK and Europe.*)

Parenteral opiates (meperidine IM and methadone IM) are extremely effective pain killers, but cause sedation, nausea and dizziness, and carry the risk of abuse.[55] Their use in migraine is restricted to the emergency room or other supervised settings where the sedation side-effects will not put the patient at risk and where the risk of abuse can be addressed. There is some concern in North America about the numbers of patients who attend the emergency room to obtain opiate analgesics for their headaches. In fact, use of these rescue therapies should be discouraged due to the risk of development of chronic daily headache with analgesic dependence.

Other combination medications

The combination of the hypnotic butalbital with aspirin, caffeine (and sometimes codeine) is available in some countries for the acute treatment of migraine. However, there is little clinical evidence for its effectiveness and concerns over the side-effects of sedation, overuse and associated rebound headaches, and problems with withdrawal restrict its use.[55]

Combinations of the sympathomimetic isometheptene with paracetamol (plus sometimes dichlorphenazone) were shown to be more effective than placebo for mild to moderate migraine in clinical trials.[55] These combinations were well tolerated, with some drowsiness, dizziness and nausea reported infrequently. One study showed that the combination of isometheptene, paracetamol and dichlorphenazone had similar efficacy to oral sumatriptan in the treatment of mild to moderate migraine attacks.[63]

Ergots

The mechanism of action of ergotamine and its derivatives is through a long-acting and non-specific vasoconstrictor action via 5-HT$_1$ receptors. This action constricts the cerebral arteries that are dilated during the migraine attack. However, the long duration and non-specific vasoconstrictor action on vessels in other body areas leads to unwanted side-effects.[64] Ergots are contraindicated in patients with evidence of cardiovascular disease owing to the risk of myocardial ischaemia and infarction.

Ergotamine

Ergotamine has been used for many years as an acute treatment for moderate to severe migraine, sometimes in combination with caffeine or caffeine, pentobarbital and belladonna alkaloids. It can be taken orally, by subcutaneous or intramuscular injection or by suppositories. Many studies have investigated the clinical profile of ergotamine and its derivatives. However, due to its age, these studies often did not use modern dosing strategies and outcome measures. Overall, evidence of ergotamine's efficacy is inconsistent, with some studies finding no effect over placebo and others finding large differences favouring ergotamine.[55] Comparative studies have shown ergotamine to be equivalent to NSAIDs and inferior to isometheptene combinations and oral sumatriptan. Ergotamine also has a sub-optimal tolerability profile. Nausea and vomiting are commonly reported as adverse events. Long-term use is associated with habituation, analgesic rebound headaches, chronic daily headache and leg ischaemia. The clinical use of ergotamine has declined dramatically in recent years, and in the UK only the combination ergotamine/cyclizine/caffeine product Migril® is now available.

Dihydroergotamine (DHE)

DHE is a derivative of ergotamine that was designed to reduce the incidence of the typical side-effects associated with ergotamine. It was developed recently and clinical studies have used modern criteria for study design, patient selection and methodology.[60] DHE is available by intravenous, subcutaneous and intramuscular injection, and as a nasal spray. Clinical trials have shown that it is an effective treatment for moderate to severe

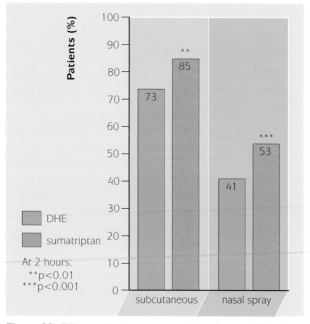

Figure 22. Efficacy of subcutaneous and nasal spray DHE at 2 hours after treatment for migraine: results of comparator trials with sumatriptan (data abstracted from references 65 and 67).

migraine (Figure 22). However, comparative trials have shown that subcutaneous and nasal spray DHE were significantly less effective than subcutaneous sumatriptan.[65,66] Nasal spray DHE was also significantly less effective than nasal spray sumatriptan.[67] However, the long duration of action of DHE results in less headache recurrence than is reported with sumatriptan. Also, DHE nasal spray was effective in preventing migraine attacks when given during the prodrome phase.[68] Although DHE has a better tolerability profile than ergotamine, nausea and vomiting are still reported and the drug is contraindicated for patients with a risk of cardiovascular disease.[55] (*DHE is currently not available for migraine in the UK.*)

Triptans

Triptans act as agonists at the 5-HT$_{1B/1D}$ receptor and have a dual mechanism of action against migraine (Figure 23):

- They have a selective vasoconstrictor action on dilated cranial blood vessels, returning them to their normal size.
- They act on trigeminal nerve terminals, reducing neuronal firing and the release of inflammatory factors.[69]

All triptans act peripherally, but are lipophilic to different extents. Some can penetrate the blood–brain barrier and hence also act significantly on central 5-HT$_1$ receptors.

Seven triptans are now available to the physician or have been approved by regulatory agencies:

Sumatriptan (Imigran®, Imitrex® in the USA and some other countries; GlaxoSmithKline) – available in oral (conventional tablet), nasal spray, subcutaneous and, in certain countries, suppository formulations.

Naratriptan (Naramig®, Amerge® in the USA; GlaxoSmithKline) – available in an oral (conventional tablet) formulation.

Zolmitriptan (Zomig®, AstraZeneca) – available in oral (conventional and orally disintegrating tablet [ODT]) formulations and submitted for regulatory approval as a nasal spray formulation.

Rizatriptan (Maxalt®; Merck, Sharp & Dohme) – available in oral (conventional and ODT) formulations.

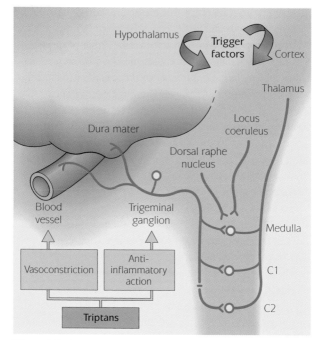

Figure 23. Mechanism of action of triptan drugs (adapted from reference 24).

Almotriptan (Almogran®, Axert® in the USA; Laboratorios Almirall) – available in an oral (conventional tablet) formulation.

Eletriptan (Relpax®; Pfizer) – approved as an oral (conventional tablet) formulation.

Frovatriptan (Elan) – recently approved by the US FDA in an oral (conventional tablet) formulation.

More triptans are still in clinical development and are likely to be introduced over the next few years, e.g. donitriptan.

Clinical profile of the triptans

All of the available triptans share many clinical features:[55]

- They are effective acute treatments for moderate to severe migraine, relieving the headache and non-headache migraine symptoms (nausea, vomiting, photophobia and phonophobia). Owing to this feature, no added anti-emetic is required.

- For oral triptans, efficacy starts within 1 hour of dosing and increases up to 2–4 hours. Typically, 60% or more of patients report headache relief by 2 hours after treatment. Nasal spray and subcutaneous formulations produce a greater response and have a more rapid onset of action. Studies suggest that administration of triptans while the pain is mild increases their efficacy.
- Triptans are effective in long-term clinical use, with about 80% of attacks being relieved at 2 hours after treatment. Efficacy in clinical practice is typically greater than that reported in controlled clinical trials.
- Headache recurrence is reported by about 30% of patients in the 24 hours following triptan dosing, necessitating a second dose. Studies demonstrate lower recurrence when migraine pain is resolved rather than just relieved.[70]
- Triptans improve the QOL of migraine patients and their use is cost-effective. Cost savings are frequently reported for triptans compared with other treatments.
- Triptans are generally well tolerated, with adverse events being characteristic of the class of drugs, including:
  - unpleasant but short-lived feelings of pain, heaviness or tightness in any part of the body, including areas such as the chest and neck, which can alarm the patient;
  - nausea;
  - drowsiness and fatigue;
  - dizziness.
- As with the ergots, there is the potential for vasoconstriction of coronary arteries, and triptans are contraindicated for patients with risk factors for cardiovascular disease. However, triptans are shorter acting than ergots, the cardiac vasoconstriction is much less and the risk of cardiovascular adverse events is low.[54] For example, sumatriptan has been shown to be well tolerated in the treatment of over 300,000 migraine attacks in clinical trials and over 200 million attacks in clinical practice. Significant cardiovascular and cerebrovascular events were only rarely reported.[71]

Pharmacological profiles of the oral triptans		
Triptan	Absorption T_{max} (h)	Plasma half-life $T_{1/2}$ (h)
Sumatriptan	2.5	2.5
Naratriptan	2–4	5.6–6.3
Zolmitriptan	2	2.5–3
Rizatriptan	1–1.5	2–3
Almotriptan	1.4–3.8	3.2–3.7
Eletriptan	1–2	3.6–5.5
Frovatriptan	2–4	25

The individual triptans have differing pharmacological properties that have been proposed to affect their clinical profile (Table 10).[72]

Sumatriptan

Sumatriptan was the first of the triptans to be developed, and has the largest portfolio of clinical data of all the triptans. It is fairly rapidly absorbed, but has low bioavailability and central nervous system penetration (Table 10).[72] It is available as 25 mg (USA only), 50 and 100 mg (not in USA) conventional tablets, 5 and 10 (USA only) and 20 mg nasal sprays, 6 mg subcutaneous injections and 12.5 and 25 mg suppositories (not in UK and USA). The clinical profile has been elucidated for all four formulations.

Oral sumatriptan

Controlled clinical trials have shown that all oral doses of sumatriptan were significantly superior to placebo for the acute treatment of migraine.[55] The proportion of patients who reported headache relief (severe or moderate headache improving to mild or none after 2 hours) were 56–62% for the 100 mg, 50–61% for the 50 mg and 52% for the 25 mg doses (Figure 24).[72] In a comparison study of the three doses, the 50 and 100 mg doses were equivalent in efficacy for moderate to severe headache, and significantly superior to the 25 mg dose.[73]

	Bioavailability (%)
	15
	63–74
	40–48
	45
	70
	50
	24–30

Table 10. Pharmacological profiles of the oral triptans. Of the triptans shown, sumatriptan penetrates the central nervous system (CNS) to the least extent (adapted from reference 72).

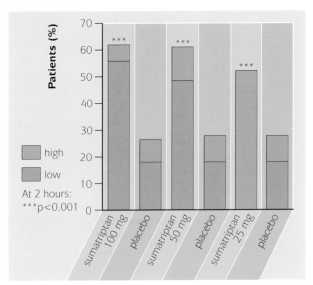

Figure 24. Efficacy of oral sumatriptan (25, 50 and 100 mg) at 2 hours after treatment for migraine (data abstracted from reference 72).

A comparator clinical study showed that sumatriptan (100 mg) was significantly superior to oral Cafergot® (ergotamine plus caffeine).[74] However, comparisons with analgesic combination medications were more equivocal. One study with aspirin plus metoclopramide showed that sumatriptan (100 mg) was superior,[75] but a second study with aspirin plus metoclopramide[76] and a study with rapid-release tolfenamic acid[77] showed no significant differences between the treatments.

Recent studies have demonstrated that migraine sufferers with significant migraine-related disability have multiple clinical presentations of their migraine attacks and that the entire spectrum of this headache activity is responsive to oral sumatriptan (50 mg).[78] In addition, intervention in a migraine attack during the mild headache phase significantly improves efficacy and reduces headache recurrence.[57] Finally, these studies suggest that disabling episodic tension-type headache is uncommon in clinical practice and that migraines, while they may begin with mild symptoms, very frequently evolve into moderate to severe headache.[31]

Nasal spray sumatriptan

Controlled clinical trials have shown that 5, 10 and 20 mg doses of sumatriptan nasal spray were significantly superior to placebo for the acute treatment of migraine.[55] The 20 mg dose was optimal, with 55–64% of patients reporting headache relief after 2 hours (Figure 25).[72] The overall response to sumatriptan nasal spray is similar to that for the oral formulation, but there is a faster onset of action (within 15 minutes of treatment).[79,80] Nasal spray sumatriptan (20 mg) was significantly more effective than nasal spray DHE.[67] The most frequently reported adverse event following sumatriptan nasal spray was a taste disturbance caused by the bitterness of the formulation. Nasal spray sumatriptan was shown to be an effective treatment for migraine attacks in adolescents and younger children (aged 5–12 years), who tend to be resistant to triptan therapy.[81,82]

Subcutaneous sumatriptan

Controlled clinical trials have shown that subcutaneous sumatriptan (6 mg) was significantly superior to placebo for the acute treatment of migraine,[55] with 81–82% of patients reporting headache relief after 2 hours (Figure 26).[72] There was a very fast onset of action, within 10 minutes of treatment. Subcutaneous

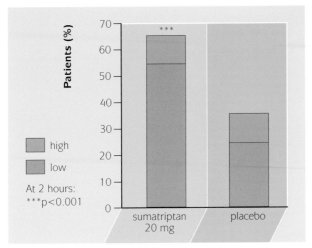

Figure 25. Efficacy of nasal spray sumatriptan (20 mg) at 2 hours after treatment for migraine (data abstracted from reference 72).

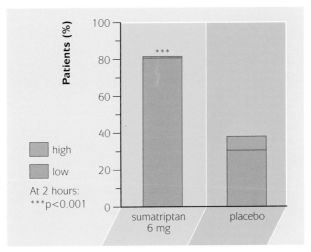

Figure 26. Efficacy of subcutaneous sumatriptan (6 mg) at 2 hours after treatment for migraine (data abstracted from reference 72).

sumatriptan is clearly the most effective of all the triptan formulations. Studies have shown it to be superior to oral

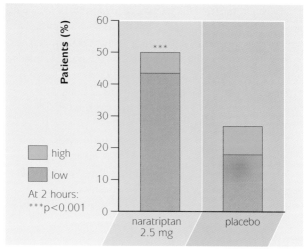

Figure 27. Efficacy of oral naratriptan (2.5 mg) at 2 hours after treatment for migraine (data abstracted from reference 72).

sumatriptan[83,84] and to subcutaneous and nasal spray DHE.[65,66] However, more adverse events were reported with subcutaneous sumatriptan than with oral triptans, especially injection site reactions, flushing, dizziness/vertigo and paraesthesia/tingling.[55]

Naratriptan

Naratriptan has a longer half-life and much higher oral bioavailability than most other triptans (Table 10), which may promote a more sustained effect.[72] It is available as a 2.5 mg conventional tablet.

Naratriptan was shown to be significantly superior to placebo as an acute treatment for migraine.[55] At first glance, naratriptan appears to be one of the least effective of the triptans, with 43–50% of patients reporting headache relief 2 hours after treatment (Figure 27).[72] However, its full efficacy is not reported until 4 hours, when 60–68% of patients reported headache relief.[85,86] The efficacy of naratriptan was maintained over a 24-hour period following treatment and it has one of the lowest reported recurrence rates of any triptan (19–28%).[72] Naratriptan is very well tolerated, with the profile of adverse events being similar to that reported for placebo.[87]

Owing to its long action, naratriptan has been investigated as a preventative or prophylactic drug for several headache subtypes. Studies have shown that it was effective for:

- The prophylaxis of transformed migraine (a type of chronic daily headache) when given at a dose of 2.5 mg/day.[88]
- The short-term prophylaxis of menstrually associated migraine when given at a dose of 1 mg twice daily.[89]
- The prevention of migraine when given at a dose of 2.5 mg during the prodrome phase of the attack.[90]
- The prophylactic treatment of cluster headache.[91]

Zolmitriptan

Zolmitriptan is absorbed rapidly and has a high bioavailability. It is more lipophilic than sumatriptan and penetrates the central nervous system to a significant extent (Table 10).[72] It is available as 2.5 mg conventional and orally disintegrating tablets (ODT), and approved as a 5 mg nasal spray. Patients take a single 2.5 mg tablet to treat their attacks, but can increase the dose to 5 mg for subsequent attacks if this dose is not effective.

Zolmitriptan was shown to be significantly superior to placebo for the acute treatment of migraine, with an onset of action within 1 hour of administration.[55] For the conventional tablet, the efficacy of the two doses was similar in clinical trials, with 62–65% of patients receiving the 2.5 mg dose and 59–67% of those receiving the 5 mg dose reporting headache relief 2 hours after treatment (Figure 28).[72] However, more adverse events were reported following the 5 mg dose. The 2.5 mg dose was also effective in treating menstrually associated attacks[92] and attacks in adolescent migraine sufferers.[93]

The 2.5 mg ODT formulation of zolmitriptan is a non-friable orange-flavoured tablet. This formulation was shown to have a similar clinical profile to the conventional tablet. A total of 63% of patients reported headache relief after 2 hours, with an onset of action within 1 hour (Figure 28). The majority of patients (70%) preferred the ODT to the conventional tablet.

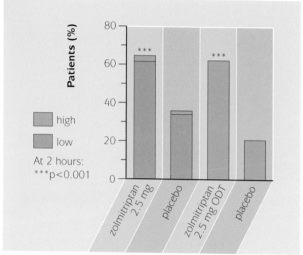

Figure 28. Efficacy of oral zolmitriptan (2.5 mg, conventional and orally disintegrating tablets) at 2 hours after treatment for migraine (data abstracted from references 72 and 94).

The ODT formulation was well tolerated, with an adverse event profile similar to that of the conventional tablet.[94]

Zolmitriptan nasal spray was apparently more effective than the oral formulations when used at a dose of 5 mg. A total of 70% of patients reported headache relief after 2 hours, with an onset of action within 15 minutes (Figure 29). The formulation was well tolerated in long-term use.[95]

Rizatriptan

Rizatriptan is a potent and selective 5-HT$_{1B/1D}$ receptor agonist that, like zolmitriptan, can act centrally as well as peripherally on receptors. It has a relatively high oral bioavailability and is rapidly absorbed (Table 10).[72] Rizatriptan is available as 5 and 10 mg conventional tablets, and as a 10 mg wafer (ODT) that dissolves on the tongue. The recommended dose is 10 mg, with a maximum of two doses in a 24-hour period.

Rizatriptan was shown to be significantly superior to placebo for the acute treatment of migraine, with an onset of action

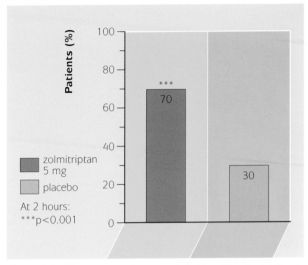

Figure 29. Efficacy of nasal spray zolmitriptan (5 mg) at 2 hours after treatment for migraine (data abstracted from reference 95).

within 30 minutes of administration.[55] For the conventional tablet, the 5 mg dose was less effective than the 10 mg dose in clinical trials, with 60–63% of patients receiving the 5 mg dose and 67–77% of those receiving the 10 mg dose reporting headache relief 2 hours after treatment (Figure 30).[72]

The rizatriptan wafer formulation is rather friable, with a mint flavour. It was shown to have a similar clinical profile to the conventional tablet. A total of 66% of patients receiving the 5 mg dose and 74% of those receiving the 10 mg dose reported headache relief at 2 hours (Figure 30).[72] Both formulations of rizatriptan were generally well tolerated in clinical trials.

Almotriptan

Almotriptan is a highly specific $5\text{-HT}_{1B/1D}$ receptor agonist with a high oral bioavailability, which acts selectively on blood vessels in the brain (Table 10).[72] It is available as a 12.5 mg conventional tablet. The recommended dose regimen is one tablet, with a maximum of two doses in a 24-hour period.

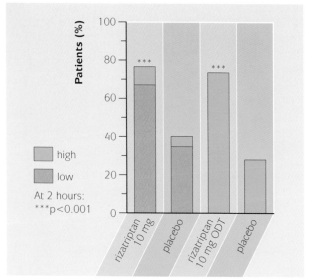

Figure 30. Efficacy of oral rizatriptan (10 mg, conventional and orally disintegrating tablets) at 2 hours after treatment for migraine (data abstracted from reference 72).

Clinical studies showed that oral almotriptan exhibited good efficacy and tolerability, and low recurrence, in the acute treatment of migraine attacks (Figure 31). A total of 64% of patients reported headache relief at 2 hours in a meta-analysis of four double-blind, controlled studies.[96] Almotriptan was well tolerated in clinical trials, with an adverse event profile similar to placebo and few chest symptoms being reported.[97]

Eletriptan

Eletriptan is an oral 5-HT$_{1B/1D}$ receptor agonist with high potency and oral bioavailability, which is selective for intracranial blood vessels over extracranial vessels (Table 10).[72,98] It is approved as 20, 40 and 80 mg conventional tablets.

Eletriptan was shown to be significantly superior to placebo for the acute treatment of migraine, with an onset of action within 30 minutes of administration.[98] In controlled clinical trials, 64–65% of patients receiving eletriptan (40 mg) reported

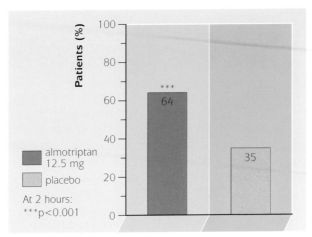

Figure 31. Efficacy of oral almotriptan (12.5 mg) at 2 hours after treatment for migraine (data abstracted from reference 96).

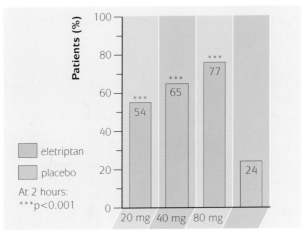

Figure 32. Efficacy of oral eletriptan at 2 hours after treatment for migraine (data abstracted from reference 99).

headache relief at 2 hours after treatment (Figure 32).[98,99] Eletriptan is generally well tolerated, although there have been some safety issues concerning elevated liver enzymes that have delayed its launch.

Frovatriptan

Frovatriptan has a high affinity for the serotonin 5-HT_{1B} and 5-HT_{1D} receptors, and is a potent stimulator of vasoconstriction in human basilar arteries. Like naratriptan, it has a long half-life, of 25 hours, but a relatively low bioavailability (Table 10).[72,100] It has been approved for the acute treatment of migraine by the FDA in the USA at an oral dose of 2.5 mg.

Frovatriptan (2.5 mg) was shown to be significantly superior to placebo for the acute treatment of migraine, but had a slow onset of action (>2.5 hours). Similar to naratriptan, the headache response following frovatriptan was not optimal at 2 hours after treatment, but increased up to 4 hours. In three controlled clinical trials, 36–46% of patients responded to frovatriptan (2.5 mg) after 2 hours and 56–65% responded after 4 hours (Figure 33).[101] Frovatriptan was generally well tolerated in these studies, with an adverse event incidence only slightly greater than that reported with placebo.[100]

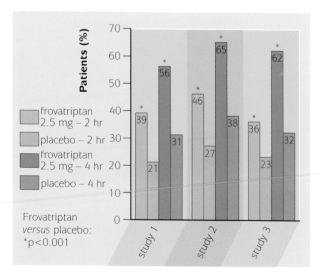

Figure 33. Efficacy of oral frovatriptan (2.5 mg) at 2 and 4 hours after treatment for migraine (data abstracted from reference 101).

Comparing the clinical profiles of the different triptans

Relatively few controlled trials have compared the clinical profiles of the different triptans, and most of these compare the newer oral drugs with the gold standard of oral sumatriptan.[98,99,102–112] However, there is intense pressure from the individual manufacturers to attempt to place their triptan in an advantageous position relative to the others. This has led to many *post hoc* analyses of clinical data, which do not provide conclusive evidence of superiority, but only suggest future avenues for research.

The overall conclusion that can be made from these studies is that no one triptan is substantially superior to another. There is also considerable debate about issues of study design, marketing spin and encapsulation of certain formulations that reduce the clinical utility of the study results.[113] A meta-analysis comparing the triptans was recently published, but again, showed only small differences, and many headache experts believe it to be flawed methodologically.[114] Since patients are treated on an individual basis, the more important question is not which triptan is best relative to another, but whether the triptan given to the patient provides the outcome desired by the patient and healthcare provider.

Perspective on the clinical profile of the triptans

The clinical profiles of the different triptans are summarized in Table 11.[72] It needs to be recognized that all the triptans are effective and well-tolerated acute treatments for moderate to severe migraine. The most effective triptan is subcutaneous sumatriptan (6 mg), which has the greatest 2-hour efficacy and fastest onset of action. Following this, the nasal spray triptans, sumatriptan (20 mg) and zolmitriptan (5 mg), have a faster onset of action and possibly slightly greater efficacy than any of the oral formulations. There seem to be only minor differences in the clinical profiles of the oral triptans. Interestingly, the clinical profiles of the ODT formulations of zolmitriptan and rizatriptan are similar to those of the equivalent conventional tablets. At present, there are no clear data to recommend one oral triptan over another. Also, the efficacy of

Summary of the clinical profiles of the different triptans from randomized, placebo-controlled clinical trials

Triptan	Dose and route of administration	ARR (%)
Sumatriptan	6 mg subcutaneous	81–82
Sumatriptan	100 mg oral	56–62
Sumatriptan	50 mg oral	50–61
Sumatriptan	25 mg oral	52
Sumatriptan	20 mg nasal spray	55–64
Naratriptan	2.5 mg oral	43–50
Zolmitriptan	2.5 mg oral	62–65
Zolmitriptan	2.5 mg ODT	63
Zolmitriptan	5 mg nasal spray	70
Rizatriptan	10 mg oral	67–77
Rizatriptan	10 mg ODT	74
Almotriptan	12.5 mg oral	64
Eletriptan	40 mg oral	65
Frovatriptan	2.5 mg oral	36–46

ARR = triptan response rate; PRR = placebo response rate (percentage of patients who improved from severe or moderate headache pain to mild or none 2 hours after treatment);

Table 11. Summary of the clinical profiles of the different triptans from randomized, placebo-controlled clinical trials (data abstracted from references 72, 94, 95, 96, 99 and 101).

a drug as assessed in clinical trials does not necessarily echo its profile in clinical practice. This has been recognized by the FDA, who require the statement "Comparisons of drug performance based on results obtained in different clinical trials are never reliable" on most triptan labels. Rather, an evaluation of each patient as to their clinical needs and desires should drive the choice of triptan. The factors that should be considered by the physician in prescribing specific triptans are explored in detail in the next section.

PRR (%)	TG (%)	NNT
31–39	43–50	2.0–2.3
17–26	30–40	2.5–3.3
17–27	24–37	2.7–4.2
17–27	25–35	2.9–4.0
25–36	24–39	2.6–4.2
18–27	16–28	3.6–6.3
34–36	25–31	3.2–3.8
22	41	2.4
30	40	2.5
35–40	27–40	2.5–3.7
28	46	2.2
35	29	3.4
24	41	2.4
21–27	9–25	4.0–11.1

TG = therapeutic gain (ARR minus PRR); NNT = number needed to treat (the number of patients it is necessary to treat to achieve one patient with a successful response, adjusted for placebo)

Prophylactic treatments for migraine

Migraine prophylaxis is worth considering if the patient suffers from more than three to four attacks per month, sufferers from concomitant co-morbidities, or a medical illness that precludes effective acute therapy. However, frequent migraine attacks may also be an indicator for chronic daily headache. Efficacy for prophylactic drugs is defined as a reduction in migraine frequency of >50%.[115] Although the "ideal" prophylactic would abolish migraine attacks altogether, in clinical trials only a maximum of about half of patients respond to this extent. Patients therefore need to have an effective acute treatment available for the inevitable breakthrough attacks that occur. The main prophylactic agents available are beta-blockers, 5-HT$_2$ antagonists, calcium antagonists, tricyclic antidepressants, selective serotonin re-uptake inhibitors (SSRIs) and sodium valproate, although not all of these medications are available in all countries. In recent years, the use of migraine prophylaxis has fallen due to the increased availability of effective acute medications, such as the triptans.

Beta-blockers

The beta-blockers propranolol, atenolol, metoprolol and timolol have been shown to be effective in migraine prophylaxis. Placebo-controlled studies showed that propranolol was significantly superior to placebo, with 35–60% of patients receiving propranolol reporting ≥50% reduction in migraine attack frequency (Figure 34).[116–119] However, propranolol had little effect on reducing the severity or duration of the breakthrough attacks that occurred.[117,120] The side-effects of beta-blockers include arterial hypotension, muscle fatigue, violent dreams, weight gain, bronchospasm and impotence.[115]

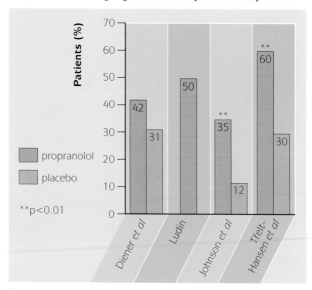

Figure 34. Efficacy of the beta-blocker propranolol for migraine prophylaxis: proportion of patients with a ≥50% reduction in migraine attack frequency (data abstracted from references 116–119).

5-HT$_2$ antagonists

Pizotifen (*not available in the USA*) and methysergide have been shown to be significantly more effective than placebo in migraine prophylaxis, but have a high frequency of side-effects. Controlled trials have shown that pizotifen reduces attack frequency by ≥50% in 35–50% of patients (Figure 35).[121–127] As with beta-blockers, pizotifen had little effect on the initial severity of breakthrough attacks.[128] The most common side-effects are drowsiness and increased appetite, which leads to significant weight gain in about 40% of patients. When weight gain occurs, it can limit compliance in what is a primarily female patient population.[129]

Lisuride is used in some countries for migraine prophylaxis, although there is little evidence for its efficacy.[115]

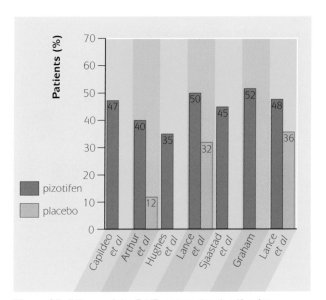

Figure 35. Efficacy of the 5-HT$_2$ antagonist pizotifen for migraine prophylaxis: proportion of patients with a ≥50% reduction in migraine attack frequency (data abstracted from references 121–127).

Calcium antagonists

Flunarizine (*not available in the UK and the USA*) has been shown to be significantly more effective than placebo in migraine prophylaxis and has efficacy similar to the beta-blocker metoprolol in a clinical trial.[130] However, there is the potential for significant side-effects with the use of these drugs, such as sedation, weight gain, depression and extrapyramidal symptoms (tremor and Parkinsonism),[115] and their availability is limited to certain countries only.

Other prophylactic drugs

The antidepressant amitriptyline is used for the prophylaxis of migraine and other headaches, particularly chronic tension-type headache and chronic daily headache (see pp. 83, 85). Although there are relatively few clinical trials of this drug showing it to be effective in migraine headache prophylaxis,[131–134] it has proved useful in clinical practice. However, side-effects include dry mouth, arterial hypotension, urinary retention, sedation and akathisia.[115]

Recent clinical trials have shown that the anticonvulsant, sodium valproate, is an effective migraine prophylactic agent, with an efficacy profile similar to that of the beta-blockers. Controlled trials have shown that sodium valproate reduced attack frequency by ≥50% in 45–50% of patients (Figure 36).[135–137] Sodium valproate was generally well tolerated, the most frequently reported adverse events being mild to moderate nausea, asthenia, dyspepsia, dizziness, somnolence and diarrhoea.[138] Women of child-bearing potential should avoid pregnancy while on sodium valproate: it reduces fertility and increases the risk of foetal abnormalities in the first trimester of pregnancy.

DHE is used as a prophylactic in certain European countries, even though there are few clinical data to support its use. Also, daily use of DHE can lead to the development of chronic daily headache.[115]

Aspirin and NSAIDs (especially naproxen) show some evidence of efficacy in migraine prophylaxis, although their gastrointestinal side-effects limit the chronic use of these drugs.[115]

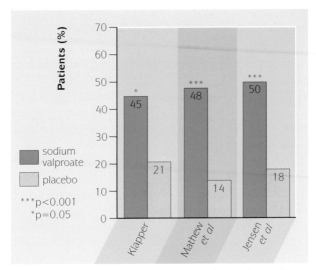

Figure 36. Efficacy of the anticonvulsant sodium valproate for migraine prophylaxis: proportion of patients with a ≥50% reduction in migraine attack frequency (data abstracted from references 135–137).

Perspective on the clinical profile of migraine prophylactic drugs

Drugs with proven efficacy for migraine prophylaxis that can be used as first-line therapies include:

- The beta-blockers propranolol and metoprolol.
- The calcium antagonist flunarizine.
- The anticonvulsant sodium valproate.

Drugs that are effective, but without large double-blind, placebo-controlled clinical trials demonstrating their efficacy, or that have serious side-effects that limit their use, include:

- The 5-HT$_2$ antagonists pizotifen, methysergide and lisuride.
- DHE.
- Aspirin and NSAIDs.
- The antidepressant amitriptyline (although this is commonly used for chronic daily headache – see p. 85).

Alternative treatments for migraine

Many migraine sufferers are attracted to alternative treatments for their migraine, for a variety of reasons:

- Exhaustion of conventional options.
- Fashion.
- The therapist gives them more time than their physician does.
- A feeling that these therapies offer them a greater level of individual control.
- An assumption that these therapies are more "natural" and safe.

  Alternative treatments used fall into two categories:

- Alternative prophylactic therapies.
- Behavioural therapies.

Alternative prophylactic therapies

Treatments that sufferers can buy OTC or in health food shops in an attempt to reduce the frequency of their migraine headaches include feverfew, homeopathic remedies, riboflavin and magnesium. Some patients try the non-pharmacological intervention of acupuncture.

Feverfew

Two clinical studies have indicated that feverfew (*Tanacetum parthenium*) may be effective as migraine prophylaxis. One study showed a reduction in attack frequency and severity with feverfew compared with placebo,[139] and the other showed an increase in the frequency and severity of attacks when feverfew treatment was stopped in patients taking the treatment.[140] However, feverfew should be used with caution, as its safety profile has not been evaluated in controlled clinical trials and commercial preparations differ widely in the concentration of active ingredient.

Homeopathic remedies

Evidence for the utility of homeopathic remedies in migraine is limited to two conflicting clinical trials. One randomized, double-blind study indicated that homeopathic treatment was no better than placebo.[141] The second study, although showing that homeopathic medications reduced the frequency of migraine attacks, did not select migraine patients on the basis of the IHS diagnostic criteria,[1] which raises questions as to the validity of the patient population studied.[142]

Riboflavin

The brains of migraine sufferers may have reduced mitochondrial energy metabolism compared with people without migraine. The rationale for using riboflavin as a migraine prophylactic agent is that it has the potential to increase mitochondrial energy efficiency.[143] A single controlled clinical trial has shown that high-dose riboflavin was significantly more effective than placebo in migraine prophylaxis. Riboflavin reduced attack frequency by ≥50% in 59% of patients compared with 15% for placebo (p<0.01) and was well tolerated.[144] However, further studies are required to confirm these data before riboflavin can be recommended for clinical use.

Magnesium

Brain magnesium levels are low during the migraine attack, which may affect migraine-related receptors and neurotransmitters.[145] The daily supplementation of magnesium may theoretically replace this magnesium and therefore prevent migraine attacks. Two controlled clinical trials have shown that chronic oral supplementation of magnesium significantly reduced the frequency of migraine attacks compared with placebo.[146,147] However, a third study showed no benefit over placebo in terms of reducing attack frequency by ≥50%, the recognized standard for efficacy.[148] More studies are therefore required before magnesium can be added to the armamentarium of clinically proven migraine prophylactic agents.

Acupuncture

A systematic, evidence-based review has recently been published on the effectiveness of acupuncture in primary headaches.[149] Of the 16 trials comparing true acupuncture with "sham" acupuncture in migraine and tension-type headache:

- Eight trials showed true acupuncture to be significantly superior.
- Four trials showed a trend in favour of true acupuncture.
- Two trials showed no difference between the treatments.
- Two trials were uninterpretable.

This evidence supports the value of acupuncture as a treatment for migraine and tension-type headache. However, larger and more rigorous trials are required to determine the true place of acupuncture in migraine therapy.

Behavioural therapies
Biofeedback and relaxation
Biofeedback is the process of bringing involuntary physiological functions under voluntary control. Biofeedback trains the nervous system to shut out excessive stimulation through calming music, visualization and slow diaphragmatic breathing.[5] Several studies support the use of biofeedback to prevent migraine attacks.[150] However, relaxation therapy may be equally as effective as biofeedback.[151] Relaxation therapy is a simple technique that can be taught by any healthcare provider. It can be practised in groups without special equipment, and is less costly and time-consuming than any biofeedback technique.[32]

Other behavioural therapies
Other behavioural approaches to migraine therapy that may prove useful to patients include:

- Development of coping skills.
- Cognitive restructuring, converting negative thoughts into positive messages.
- Assertiveness training.
- Goal identification.
- Manipulative procedures.
- Massage.
- Exercise – a routine of 20–40 minutes aerobic exercise per day.[5]

Many of these techniques help to reduce stress, which is one of the major trigger factors for migraine (see pp. 28–29).

Perspective on the clinical profile of migraine alternative therapies

Of the alternative therapies evaluated for migraine, the following have clinical evidence of efficacy and may therefore be recommended by the physician:

- Biofeedback and/or relaxation therapies.
- Magnesium prophylaxis.
- Riboflavin prophylaxis.
- Feverfew prophylaxis.
- Acupuncture prophylaxis.

The patient needs to decide which, if any, of these therapies appeals to them, is affordable or practicable to their lifestyles.

Treatments for other headache types

Tension-type headache

Since acute tension-type headache produces little impact and is readily managed by most people outside the healthcare system, as a single entity it is not commonly encountered in medical practice. It is, however, frequently seen as part of the headache spectrum in those with migraine. In this setting, based on its response to migraine-specific medication, many consider it to be pathophysiologically similar to migraine. In fact, it has been suggested that tension-type headache in migraine sufferers is a distinct entity from tension-type headache without migraine.[78]

Management of acute tension-type headache usually includes OTC medications such as aspirin, paracetamol and NSAIDs, and non-drug approaches such as relaxation, hot baths and massage. These treatments are usually effective and further intervention is rarely necessary. Management of chronic tension-type headache is more complex and is dealt with below under "Chronic daily headaches", but amitriptyline has been shown to be effective as prophylaxis.[152,153] Unlike dothiepin, amitriptyline has no associated risk for developing ischaemic heart disease.[154]

Short, sharp headache

Owing to the short duration of these headaches, acute treatments tend to be of little use and reassurance that these headaches are benign is usually enough. However, various prophylactic medications can be useful:

- NSAIDs taken daily, e.g. diclofenac or indomethacin.
- Sodium valproate.
- Tricyclic antidepressants, which are also used for chronic paroxysmal hemicrania.[153]

Cluster headache

Cluster headache is usually managed by neurologists or headache specialists in a specialist setting. Since cluster headache is of short duration, abortive treatment must be rapid in onset, and thus oral formulations are of limited value. Successfully used drugs include the following:[35]

- Subcutaneous sumatriptan (6 mg) is very effective against cluster headache and is the abortive treatment of choice.[155] Nasal spray sumatriptan (20 mg) is also effective.[156] However, oral triptans are relatively ineffective. Oral zolmitriptan (5 mg) has only modest efficacy against episodic cluster headache, much lower than subcutaneous sumatriptan or oxygen.[157]
- Inhalation of high-flow-rate oxygen is also effective as an abortive treatment in about 70% of patients, usually within 5–10 minutes of dosing.[158,159]
- Nasally applied lignocaine is a useful adjunct to other abortive therapies.[35]

Prophylaxis is the mainstay of cluster headache management, initiated at the beginning of a new cluster period. The following drugs have been shown to be effective:

- Corticosteroids (prednisolone), methysergide and ergotamine can be used for short-term prophylaxis. Prednisolone can provide relief for chronic cluster attacks or cover the introduction of medication at the beginning of a cluster period.
- Verapamil and lithium are used for long-term prophylaxis.[35]

Chronic daily headache

Cases of chronic daily headache are usually referred to neurologists or headache specialists for management.[160] There are four strategies for the management of this headache:

- Physical measures, such as physiotherapy of the neck. This is of help when the patient, as often, has a history of head or neck injury.
- Withdrawal of drugs causing rebound headaches, such as codeine and ergotamine.
- Headache prophylactic drugs, including:
  - tricyclic antidepressants, e.g. prothiaden and amitriptyline;
  - anticonvulsants, e.g. sodium valproate, gabapentin and topiramate.
- Acute medications to treat breakthrough migraine attacks, e.g. triptans.[153]

Facial pain
Sinus headache (sinusitis)

First-line therapy for sinus headache of infectious aetiology is:

- A broad-spectrum antibiotic.
- Local measures, e.g. steam inhalation or vasoconstrictor agents.
- Oral decongestants, if treatment is required for more than 72 hours.[161]

If no signs of infection are evident, and there is a history of recurrent stable episodes of headache, the diagnosis of migraine should be considered.[162] If this fails, referral to a specialist is probably required.

Trigeminal neuralgia

The first-line drug for trigeminal neuralgia is usually the anticonvulsant carbamazepine. Alternatives include other anticonvulsants (sodium valproate or gabapentin), the muscle relaxant baclofen and the benzodiazepine clonazepam. The patient can be referred for surgery if these drugs do not control the symptoms.[161]

Post-herpetic neuralgia

Three strategies are used in series to manage this condition, dependent on the stage of the illness:

- During the acute eruption of pain, the best approach to treating this condition is the use of antiviral drugs such as aciclovir or valaciclovir. There is a greatly reduced likelihood of patients developing post-herpetic pain if they take these drugs very early in the illness.[36]
- In the acute phase of the rash, analgesics are often used, together with topical applications such as camomile to reduce local irritation.
- Once the rash has cleared and a definite diagnosis of herpetic neuralgia made, tricyclic antidepressants are the mainstay of treatment, together with local application of capsaicin.[161]

Temporomandibular joint dysfunction

This condition is usually managed by a dentist, e.g. by fitting a customized gum shield for use at night. Supplementary medical strategies include stress management programmes and prophylaxis with tricyclic antidepressants.[161]

Management of Migraine in the Primary Care Setting

As described in the section on "Current Migraine Management in Primary Care", the goals of migraine management are to:

- Encourage migraine sufferers to engage with the healthcare system, to consult their primary care provider and receive appropriate treatment.
- Motivate currently consulting migraine patients to continue with their care.
- Provide physicians with simple but comprehensive guidelines to allow them to diagnose migraine differentially from other headaches.
- Encourage physicians to provide prescription medications that have been proven to be effective (Figure 37).[50]

Recently published guidelines for migraine care advocate the following management scheme:[5,54–56]

- Provide patient counselling and seek their buy-in.
- Make a careful diagnosis.
- Assess migraine impact in the initial evaluation of patients.
- Produce an individual treatment plan for each patient.
    - Patients with disabling migraine should be provided with migraine-specific therapies from the outset.
- Implement follow-up procedures to monitor the outcome of therapy.

This section describes how these concepts can be translated into a practical scheme for the management of migraine and other headaches in primary care. The first four points above need to be dealt with at the patient's initial consultation. The fifth point is dealt with at follow-up consultations. An algorithm for the management of migraine at the individual patient level is shown in Figure 38.

The first consultation

Providing patient counselling and seeking their buy-in

With most patients having a history of self-treating with OTC

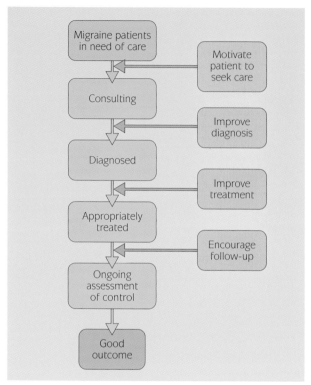

Figure 37. Goals of migraine management to improve consultation rates, diagnosis, treatment and monitoring of care (adapted from reference 164).

medications (and not always successfully), the first consultation may be the only opportunity the primary care physician has to manage the migraine effectively. Patients need to be shown that they are being listened to, and use the consultation to formulate a constructive management plan. This will demonstrate to them that they are being well managed and encourage them to return for follow-up care. It is wise to make a specific appointment to discuss the patient's headache, and to involve other members of the primary healthcare team, e.g. nurses and receptionists, to make optimum use of the time available (see pp. 107–108).

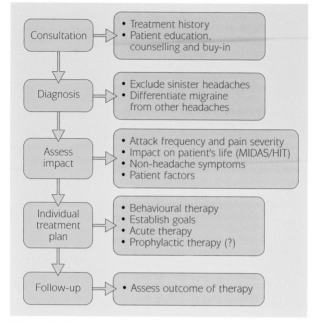

Figure 38. A proposed algorithm for individual patient management of migraine.

Taking a treatment history

Taking a headache history is key to the first consultation. Patients will already have tried OTC medications that may distort symptoms classically used in recognition and diagnosis. Patients may have also consulted a physician unsuccessfully in the past and tried prescribed therapies. The physician needs to know the patient's previous experience of headache management. In most instances, history is taken when a person is not experiencing severe headache and hence the provider is obtaining a composite picture of that person's headaches over time. Given the wide range of symptoms that can occur from migraine to migraine and the distortion of the natural evolution of a migraine that occurs with self-treatment effort, it is often best to have a patient focus first on their most problematic headache presentation. No single symptom defines migraine and thus the physician uses the history to create clinical pictures representative of the headache pattern. Ideally, the history should cover:

- Headache – the impact, type, severity, location, duration, frequency, timing and family history.
- Other symptoms – visual, sensory, gastrointestinal.
- Influencing factors – diet, lifestyle, hormonal, environmental.
- Current medication for headaches and other conditions.

An example of a headache history card is shown in Figure 39. The nurse can help the patient to complete this card before they meet the physician. Nurses will meet many patients with headache at well-person clinics, routine vaccinations, antenatal, baby and family planning clinics, and can be proactive in this area.

Patient education about their condition

Patients with a history of unsuccessful treatment may be sceptical of further medical care. They need to be shown that their physician takes migraine seriously, and that new and effective therapies are available. People with headache are often motivated to understand their condition, and physicians should provide them with information on the nature and mechanisms of their disorder. Many of the organizations listed in Appendix 2 provide leaflets about migraine and have websites that the patient can consult. Patients should be told that, even though primary headaches cannot be cured, the pain and other symptoms can be controlled and their impact minimized. An explicit understanding of realistic treatment goals can improve patient satisfaction with care.

Patient buy-in

As with other chronic conditions, patients need to manage their migraine themselves, making decisions about lifestyle alterations and how and when to take their medications. Physicians should encourage their patients to participate in their own management, and effective communication between the physician and patient has been shown to improve care

Headache History Card
Please tick the relevant box

Severity

___ Mild
___ Severe

Frequency

___ Several times a year
___ Several times a month
___ Several times a week
___ Once a year
___ Once a month
___ Once a week

Advance warning

___ Always
___ Sometimes
___ Never

What sort of warning do you get?

___ Visual disturbance
___ Numbness/tingling
___ Speech difficulties
___ Sensitivity to light
___ Feelings of weakness
___ None of the above

Where is the pain usually located?

___ Top of the head
___ Back of the head
___ One side of the head
___ Both sides of the head
___ Front of head
___ Other

How would you describe the pain?

___ An aching pain
___ A throbbing pain
___ A stabbing pain
___ A burning pain
___ None of these

Do you have any other symptoms during the headache?

___ Nausea/vomiting
___ Visual disturbance
___ Feelings of weakness
___ Speech difficulties
___ Loss of appetite
___ Dizziness
___ Sensitivity to light/noise
___ Numbness/tingling

Is the headache so bad you have to go to bed?

___ Always
___ Sometimes
___ Never

How long does your headache last?

___ Less than one hour
___ One to four hours
___ Four to six hours
___ Six to 12 hours
___ 12 to 24 hours
___ More than 24 hours

Figure 39. Example of a headache history card. Reprinted with permission from reference 32; copyright MIPCA, 1998).

delivery.[163] Patient preference is an important consideration in the choice of treatment. Patients may rate such factors as speed of response, overall headache relief, lack of side-effects or convenience as the most important characteristics of treatment.

Making a careful diagnosis

Although serious secondary headaches are rare, it must be stressed that an accurate diagnosis is essential to facilitate the successful management of migraine and other headaches in primary care. Headache diagnosis is covered in the "Diagnosis" section of this book and the physician is referred there for the necessary information. Using these criteria, diagnosis of migraine should be rapid and accurate. Additionally, it is often worth asking the patient what self-diagnosis they would give!

Assessing migraine impact in the initial evaluation of patients

The physician needs to assess the patient's illness severity in order to select an appropriate medication. However, this is not as easy as it sounds. While pain intensity is the most important aspect of migraine to the individual sufferer and most patients consulting their physicians do so for pain relief,[39] economic studies have shown that headache-related disability is the most important determinant of migraine's societal impact in economic terms.[164] The new guidelines for migraine care recommend that the physician assesses the following criteria to determine illness severity:

- Attack frequency and pain severity.
- The impact (disability) on the patient's life.
- Associated non-headache symptoms.
- Patient factors, such as their response to prior medications, their preferences and their co-morbid illnesses.

Assessments of migraine impact have proved to be accurate measures of headache illness severity and two tools have been developed to assess this: the Migraine Disability Assessment (MIDAS) Questionnaire and the Headache Impact Test (HIT).

MIDAS is a paper-based questionnaire, designed to be accessible at physicians' surgeries and pharmacies. Migraine sufferers answer five disability questions in three activity domains covering the previous 3-month period (Figure 40).[165]

Do You Suffer From

headaches?

MIDAS QUESTIONNAIRE

INSTRUCTIONS: Please answer the following questions about ALL your headaches you have had over the last 3 months. Write your answer in the box next to each question. Write zero if you did not do the activity in the last 3 months.

1 On how many days in the last 3 months did you miss work or school because of your headaches? ☐☐ days

2 How many days in the last 3 months was your productivity at work or school reduced by half or more because of your headaches? *(Do not include days you counted in question 1 where you missed work or school)* ☐☐ days

3 On how many days in the last 3 months did you not do household work because of your headaches? ☐☐ days

4 How many days in the last 3 months was your productivity in household work reduced by half or more because of your headaches? *(Do not include days you counted in question 3 where you did not do household work)* ☐☐ days

5 On how many days in the last 3 months did you miss family, social or leisure activities because of your headaches? ☐☐ days

TOTAL ☐☐ days

A On how many days in the last 3 months did you have a headache? *(If a headache lasted more than 1 day, count each day)* ☐☐ days

B On a scale of 0–10, on average how painful were these headaches? *(Where 0 = no pain at all, and 10 = pain as bad as it can be)* ☐

©Innovative Medical Research 1997

Once you have filled in the questionnaire, add up the total number of days from questions 1–5 (ignore A and B).

Grading system for the MIDAS Questionnaire:		
Grade	Definition	Score
I	Little or no disability	0–5
II	Mild disability	6–10
III	Moderate disability	11–20
IV	Severe disability	21+

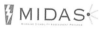

MIDAS is supported by an unrestricted educational grant from

Figure 40. The Migraine Disability Assessment (MIDAS) Questionnaire.[165] THe MIDAS programme was developed by Innovative Medical Research Inc.; with sponsorship and assistance from AstraZeneca.

They score the number of lost days due to headache in employment, household work, and family and social activities. Sufferers also report the number of additional days with significant limitations to activity (defined as at least 50% reduced productivity) in the employment and household work domains. The total MIDAS score is obtained by summing the answers to the five questions as lost days due to headache. This can sometimes be higher than the actual number of lost headache days due to any one day being counted in more than one domain. The score is categorized into four severity grades:

- Grade I = 0–5 (defined as minimal or infrequent disability).
- Grade II = 6–10 (mild or infrequent disability).
- Grade III = 11–20 (moderate disability).
- Grade IV = 21 and over (severe disability).

Two other questions (A and B) are not scored, but were designed to provide the physician with clinically relevant information on headache frequency and pain intensity. Information on MIDAS can be accessed at www.migraine-disability.net

The HIT was first developed as a web-based test, designed to be accessible to all physicians and headache sufferers through the Internet (at www.headachetest.com and www.amIhealthy.com). This is a dynamic questionnaire (Figure 41), with items derived from four validated headache questionnaires sampling all areas of headache impact.[166] Patients are questioned until clinical standards of score precision are met. In practice, five questions are sufficient to grade the majority of headache sufferers with severe, moderate or mild headache. Internet-HIT differentiates sufferers on the basis of diagnosis and characteristics such as headache severity and frequency, and takes only 1–2 minutes to complete.[167]

HIT-6 is a paper-based, short-form questionnaire based on the Internet-HIT question pool, designed for people without access to the Internet (Figure 42). Six questions cover pain severity, loss of work and recreational activities, tiredness, mood alterations and cognition. Each question is scored on a

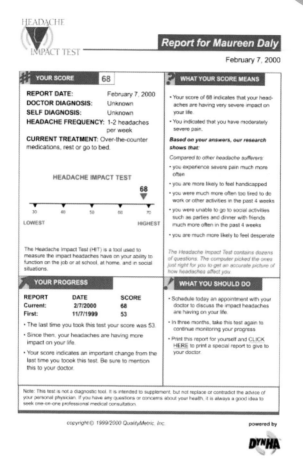

Figure 41. The Internet-HIT Questionnaire.[166] HIT was developed by Quality Metric Inc. and GlaxoSmithKline.

five-point scale, with the scores being added to produce the final score.[168] HIT-6 scores are categorized into four grades, representing minimal, mild, moderate and severe impact due to headache. Internet-HIT and HIT-6 scores compared well

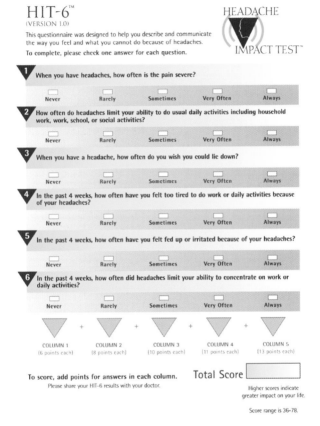

Figure 42. The HIT-6 Questionnaire.[167] HIT was developed by Quality Metric Inc. and GlaxoSmithKline.

with each other when the two forms of the questionnaire were tested on a group of headache sufferers.[167]

MIDAS and HIT have both been tested extensively and shown to be reliable and valid, with wide potential for clinical utility. They can be used to:

* Improve communication between patients and their physicians on the impact of migraine.
* Help the physician to assess illness severity.

- Help the physician to produce an individualized treatment plan for each patient, when used with other clinical assessments.
- Provide an outcome measure to monitor the success of interventions (so far demonstrated for MIDAS only).[167]

Both MIDAS and HIT were developed to assess the whole spectrum of headache, and are not restricted to migraine only. They are widely used by specialist physicians, but have had limited uptake in primary care. We encourage primary care physicians to use these tools to evaluate their patients. Patients should be encouraged to complete the forms before they see the physician, with help if needed from the receptionist or nurse at the surgery.

In addition to using the MIDAS or HIT assessment tools, it is often valuable to ask the patient to explain their expectations of headache management. Occasionally, patients may have infrequent high-impact migraines. In these cases, the impact measures will not necessarily measure the true impact of the migraine to the individual patient and thus sole reliance on these measures is not recommended.

Producing an individual treatment plan for each patient
Owing to its inherent heterogeneity,[8] migraine management needs to be tailored to each patient's individual needs. The following factors should be taken into consideration:
- Headache frequency.
- Headache duration and severity.
- Presence and severity of non-headache-associated symptoms.
- Impact of headache on the patient's life, assessed with MIDAS or HIT.
- The patient's history and preference.

Behavioural therapy
Behavioural preventative strategies should be provided for every patient. This can include relaxation or biofeedback, and advice on trigger avoidance. About 20% of patients can reduce the frequency of their migraine attacks by identifying specific

migraine triggers (risk factors) and avoiding them.[169] However, all patients should be advised to take measures that could reduce the influence of migraine triggers:

- Eat and sleep regularly.
- Try to manage stress and find ways to relax.
- Try to avoid encountering several triggers simultaneously (e.g. don't drink red wine when under stress).

Alternative therapies should not be discouraged, as the patient may be convinced that they are of benefit. However, the physician should be aware of the potential side-effects and interactions with conventional treatments that may occur.

Decisions based on headache frequency

The physician can assess headache frequency easily from the patient history or from a completed MIDAS form (Question A).

- Patients with more than three or four migraine attacks per month should be offered prophylactic medication plus acute medication for breakthrough attacks.
  - The prophylactic medications of choice are beta-blockers, calcium antagonists (where available) and sodium valproate. Amitriptyline is also often useful.
  - Menstrual migraine is sometimes managed with oral contraceptives, given prophylactically during the peri-menstrual period.
- The physician should suspect chronic daily headache if the patient has more than 15 days of "migraine" headache per month. These patients are probably best referred to a specialist for care.
- However, the majority of patients experience infrequent attacks and require acute medication only.

Establish goals of therapy

It is important that physicians and patients share an understanding of the presenting problem and expectations of treatment. Patients may not fully understand their illness and/or may have expectations of treatment that are too high or too low. Physicians often do not define for themselves concise expectations of interventions for migraine, and instead rely on broad and often vague criteria for success. The International Headache Society has suggested for research that patients are pain free 2 hours after using an acute intervention.[170] While this stringent criterion may not be possible for every patient or with every migraine, it does set a standard by which patients and providers can judge their success. The goal of prophylactic therapy should be to reduce headache frequency by >50% or improve a co-morbid condition. Finally, in order to avoid the complications of excessive analgesic overuse, it is valuable to set limits on the quantity of acute medications being consumed. Many physicians have advocated that acute medications be taken on <2 days per week. Once the physician and patient understand the presenting problem and the goals of therapy, they can work together to expedite a formal management plan.

Choosing the optimum acute therapy

Patients with migraine often experience considerable variability in their headache presentations. They often have a spectrum of headaches, some of which are high impact and others low impact. In addition, their treatment needs can vary considerably based on the dynamics of their daily life. With these modifying factors in mind, it is valuable to divide patients into two categories, based on their assessed illness severity:

- Mild to moderate intensity, requiring non-specific therapies.
- Moderate to severe intensity, requiring migraine-specific therapies.

Patients with mild to moderate migraine have the following characteristics:

- Headaches that are almost always mild to moderate in intensity (mild headaches are not generally seen in clinical practice).
- Non-headache-associated symptoms, if present, are not severe in intensity.
- The impact of the headache on the patient's lifestyle is not significant:
  - MIDAS Grade I or II (minimal or mild disability).
  - HIT Grade 1 or 2 (minimal or mild impact).

Patients with mild to moderate migraine can be prescribed analgesics or combination therapies that have proven clinical evidence of efficacy, including:

- Aspirin and NSAIDs, used in high doses, e.g. aspirin (900 mg).
- Analgesic-antiemetic combination medications, e.g. aspirin plus metoclopramide or paracetamol plus domperidone.
- Isometheptene combination medications.

For maximal effect, the physician should advise the patient to take these medications early in the attack, while the headache is still mild in intensity. However, the physician should realize that most patients will have already tried simple analgesics before they consult their physician. The physician needs to elicit the patient's treatment history before prescribing acute medications. Those who have failed previously on simple analgesics and combination medications should be prescribed a migraine-specific medication from the outset.

Patients with moderate to severe migraine have the following characteristics:

- Headaches that frequently become moderate to severe in intensity.
- Significant non-headache-associated symptoms, which may be severe in intensity.
- The impact of the headache on the patient's lifestyle is significant:
  - MIDAS Grade III or IV (moderate or severe disability).
  - HIT Grade 3 or 4 (moderate or severe impact).

Patients with moderate to severe migraine should be prescribed from the outset migraine-specific drugs that have proven clinical evidence of efficacy. The triptans have the best clinical profile of these drugs and can be recommended for most patients. Ergotamine can no longer be recommended due to the risk of habituation and development of chronic daily headache. However, DHE can be used as an alternative to triptans, particularly where a long-acting effect is required.

All the available triptans are effective and well-tolerated treatments, but no one triptan is an unequivocal choice. However, some general principles for prescribing can be outlined:

- Triptans are effective for migraine without aura and migraine with aura, and for migraine subtypes such as menstrual migraine and early-morning migraine that is fully developed upon wakening.

- Most patients can be effectively treated with one of the oral triptans.

- If a patient is effectively managed with an established oral triptan, there is no need to introduce a new triptan because of small theoretical improvements in efficacy that may be promoted by the manufacturers.

- If one triptan fails, an alternative triptan is likely to be effective and should be prescribed.[104]

- If a patient has unpredictable migraine attacks or has difficulty in swallowing tablets during their attacks, they may prefer to use one of the ODT formulations of zolmitriptan or rizatriptan that can be taken at any time without water.

- Patients who have rapidly developing severe attacks may require a particularly fast-acting triptan. In this case, nasal spray sumatriptan or zolmitriptan, or subcutaneous sumatriptan, may be appropriate.

- Patients with severe nausea or vomiting may be unable to take oral or nasal spray triptans. In this case, subcutaneous sumatriptan should be tried.

- Patients who have difficulties in tolerating oral triptans can be given naratriptan or almotriptan, which may have fewer associated side-effects than the other triptans.[87,112]

- Patients who experience frequent headache recurrence may benefit from naratriptan or almotriptan, which have the least associated recurrence rates of any of the triptans.[102,103] Other long-acting drugs, such as DHE or frovatriptan, may also be useful.

- A self-administered rescue medication should be supplied to treat non-responders or headache recurrence. This is usually a second dose of the original triptan.

Patients should be told to take their triptan or DHE at the start of the headache phase when the headache is mild. Until recently, patients were told to take their medication when the headache was established and moderate or severe in intensity. This advice followed the study design in triptan clinical trials.[60] However, recent clinical evidence from the Spectrum Study showed that sumatriptan was most effective when given early in the attack, when the migraine headache was mild (Figure 43).[58]

Further evidence from the Spectrum Study showed that sumatriptan was effective for the range of headaches experienced by migraine sufferers, including tension-type

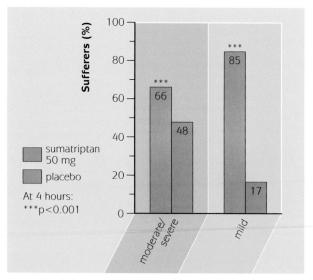

Figure 43. Efficacy of sumatriptan (50 mg) at 4 hours after treatment when given for mild or moderate/severe migraine headache (data abstracted from reference 58).

headache as well as migraine attacks (Figure 44). This indicated that triptans can be used to treat all headaches experienced by migraine sufferers, which simplifies their everyday use.[78]

Follow-up consultations

Implement follow-up procedures to monitor the outcome of therapy

Once the first consultation is over, it is important to set in place follow-up procedures to motivate patients to persevere with their treatment and return to the clinic for further care. A good way to do this is to issue a headache/migraine diary (Figure 45), asking the patient to return in a few weeks with the completed diary. A MIDAS or HIT Questionnaire can also be given out at this time. The practice nurse can issue these forms and provide guidance if necessary.

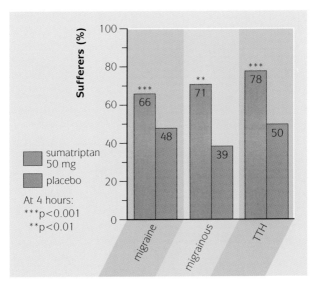

Figure 44. Efficacy of sumatriptan (50 mg) at 4 hours after treatment for the spectrum of headache experienced by migraine sufferers (migraine, migrainous headache and tension-type headache [TTH]) (data abstracted from reference 78).

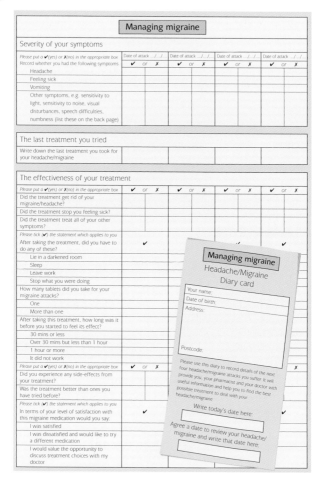

Figure 45. Example of a headache/migraine diary. Reprinted with permission from reference 32; copyright MIPCA, 1998).

At follow-up assessments, the physician can use the completed diary cards and HIT Questionnaire to confirm the diagnosis, and the diary cards and MIDAS Questionnaire to objectively assess the efficacy of treatment:[167]

- Patients who were treated effectively should continue with that therapy.

- Patients who have failed on analgesics or combination medications should be provided with migraine-specific medications, usually a triptan.
- Patients who have failed on a triptan can be provided with an alternative triptan.
- Patients who find their triptan effective, but inconvenient to use, can be provided with an alternative formulation that suits their needs better.
- Patients refractory to triptans, or who require regular rescue therapy, may require drugs such as butorphanol or codeine-containing drugs for rescue. However, due to the danger of habituation and chronic daily headache, it is probably best to refer these patients to a specialist for treatment.

Prophylaxis is not intended as a long-term management strategy, but should be reviewed after 3 months. If the treatment is effective, without causing chronic side-effects, treatment can be continued up to 6 months. If not, an alternative prophylactic drug can be supplied. At 6 months, the prophylactic can be withdrawn if the frequency of attacks is reduced. Providing the frequency remains reduced after withdrawal, it may be appropriate to revert to acute treatments only.

Patients who are refractory to repeated acute and/or prophylactic medications may need to be referred to a specialist for further care.

Management of other headaches in primary care

Secondary (sinister) headache

Patients suspected of having this headache should be evaluated thoroughly. Often this is accomplished by referral to a hospital or to a specialist, depending on the seriousness of the condition.

Tension-type headache

In spite of it being the most common headache, tension-type headache is seen relatively infrequently in primary care. Sufferers usually find OTC medications such as aspirin, paracetamol and NSAIDs effective. As we have shown, tension-type headache attacks occurring in migraine patients can be treated effectively with the triptans.[78]

Short, sharp headache

Reassurance that the symptoms of short, sharp headache are benign is usually all that patients require. Patients who demand treatment may be best referred to a specialist. However, daily NSAIDs can be provided. Indomethacin is the gold standard as it causes fewer gastrointestinal side-effects than other NSAIDs.

Cluster headache

After diagnosis, patients with cluster headache are best referred to a specialist for management. Subcutaneous sumatriptan (6 mg) is the gold standard for abortive treatment. Oxygen inhalation may also be useful if the patient has access to the necessary high-flow-rate equipment. Prophylaxis with prednisolone, methysergide or ergotamine (short term), or verapamil or lithium (long term) is also usually prescribed (see p. 84).[35]

Chronic daily headache

Management of chronic daily headache can be complex, and such cases are probably best referred to a neurologist or headache specialist following diagnosis in primary care. Management involves avoidance of analgesics, physical measures to the neck, and appropriate prophylactic and acute treatments (see p. 85).[153]

Facial pain
Sinus headache secondary to infectious aetiology

The physician can provide a broad-spectrum antibiotic and recommend steam inhalation or vasoconstrictor agents for local treatment. Oral decongestants can be provided if treatment is required for more than 72 hours. If this fails, it is probably best to refer the patient to a specialist.[161]

However, misdiagnosis is perhaps the greatest pitfall with sinus headache. A positive diagnosis of sinusitis is required.

Evidence of acute sinusitis, with a purulent discharge from the nose, and support with imaging or using a flexible scope, can confirm the diagnosis. In the absence of this evidence, migraine may be a more likely diagnosis.[162]

Trigeminal neuralgia

Following diagnosis, the physician should prescribe carbamazepine for trigeminal neuralgia. If this or alternative drugs do not control the symptoms, referral for surgery may be appropriate.[161]

Post-herpetic neuralgia

The three strategies of:

- antiviral drugs during the acute eruption of pain,
- analgesics and topical applications in the acute phase of the rash, and
- tricyclic antidepressants and local application of capsaicin once the rash has cleared
  - can be used in primary care to manage post-herpetic neuralgia.[36]

Temporomandibular joint dysfunction

This condition is usually best managed by a dentist.[161]

The primary care headache team

The management of headache in primary care is, of necessity, a long-term business. Patients need to be evaluated and treated carefully over a period of time. The physician's time and energy can be conserved during this process by using other members of the primary healthcare team.

The practice nurse can conduct much of the evaluation of the patient before they see the physician:

- Completing a headache history and MIDAS or HIT evaluation.
- Explaining about migraine and the medications used to treat it.
- Giving out and evaluating headache diary cards.

- Advocating the early use of OTC medications to be taken when the headache is mild in intensity.
- Referring appropriate patients to the physician for diagnosis and treatment.
- Helping sufferers identify possible triggers.

The nurse can meet headache patients during the course of their regular duties (opportunistically or during health screenings) or by the setting up of a dedicated headache clinic.

The community pharmacist can also be an integral part of the primary care headache team. The pharmacist is often the first source of healthcare advice that headache sufferers use and may well see the sufferer at the time of an attack. The pharmacist can:

- Educate headache sufferers about their condition.
- Identify some migraine sufferers and provide them with OTC medications that may be effective.
- Advise appropriate sufferers to consult their primary care physician.
- Encourage sufferers to go back to their physician if their current prescribed medication is not working.

With the help of these other healthcare professionals, the physician can concentrate at the first visit on:

- the accurate differential diagnosis of the headache,
- choosing medications appropriate to the patient's illness severity and lifestyle needs, or
- referring patients with sinister symptoms, cluster headache or chronic daily headache to a specialist.

At follow-up visits the physician can:

- review the progress of the patient and modify treatment if indicated, or
- refer to specialists those patients who cannot be dealt with in the primary care setting.

In the future, other primary healthcare providers who may encounter headache sufferers, e.g. school nurses, chiropractors, opticians and dentists, may be able to use these approaches to manage headache in an appropriate way.

Frequently Asked Questions: Explanations for Patients

What is migraine?

Migraine is a clinical syndrome consisting of multiple symptoms, including headache, nausea, sensory sensitivity, muscle pain, cognitive disruptions and autonomic symptoms, that occurs in an episodic fashion over decades of a sufferer's life. Genetic factors may determine the threshold for migraine sensitivity.

What are the differences between migraine and tension-type headache?

The most fundamental distinction between these headaches is the impact they create for the sufferer. From a taxonomy viewpoint, migraine is distinguished from tension-type headache by a greater number of, and more severe, symptoms, although there is significant symptom overlap. Many doctors believe that migraine and tension-type headache share similar pathophysiological mechanisms, at least in migraine sufferers. Chronic daily headache is differentiated on the frequency of the headache. It may evolve from an episodic pattern of either migraine or tension-type headache or less commonly, *de novo*.

Who is susceptible to migraine?

There is often a positive family history for both migraine and tension-type headache, and thus it appears genetic factors have a role in determining who gets headaches. Less commonly, migraine can occur after head or neck trauma, psychological trauma or infections. It therefore appears that many factors are involved in determining who gets migraine.

What causes migraine?

When a susceptible nervous system confronts a migraine-provoking environment, neurochemical changes occur, often resulting in premonitory symptoms. Eventually, a critical threshold is reached and an area in the brain stem is activated (the hypothesized "migraine generator"). The threshold for activation of sensory input is diminished and sensory symptoms emerge, for example, sensitivity to light and/or sound and odours. The emergence of muscle pain and mild headache also occur. As the process progresses, changes to brain blood vessels occur (vasodilatation and neuro-inflammation), as well as activation of autonomic nerves (leading to nausea, vomiting, diarrhoea, nasal congestion and lacrimation). If this process is not terminated, pain processing mechanisms are disrupted in the brain, the headache pain becomes severe, and pain may spread to the scalp, face and extremities (i.e. allodynia).

Is migraine caused by menstruation?

Women of reproductive years frequently experience migraine near or at the time of menses and a small proportion (14%) experience migraine only associated with their menses. Most doctors believe that migraine occurs as the oestrogen levels rapidly fall at this time. Hormonal fluctuations are more correctly thought of as a trigger or risk factor rather than as a "cause".

What are the symptoms of migraine?

The symptoms associated with an attack of migraine can vary considerably from patient to patient or attack to attack. They generally evolve over time through a predictable pattern. These can be divided into pre-headache, headache and post-headache phases. Non-localized pre-headache symptoms are called the premonitory or prodrome phase. Typical symptoms include mood changes, fatigue, muscle pain, food cravings or cognitive difficulties. In 10–15% of attacks, pre-headache symptoms may be localized and constitute aura. These are usually visual but may be sensory or, infrequently, motor. The headache phase generally begins as a mild diffuse headache that becomes localized and moderate to severe in intensity. Migraine-associated symptoms such as photophobia, phonophobia, nausea and vomiting also commonly occur. The headache phase typically lasts 4–72 hours. The post-headache phase is sometimes called the "migraine hangover". At this stage, the headache has resolved, but associated symptoms may linger for another day or two.

What are the symptoms of a tension-type headache?

Tension-type headache is a non-descript headache syndrome. It is defined more by its lack of migraine features than by its own symptomatology. The headache, typically dull and diffuse, can prohibit but not inhibit activity. There is a lack of nausea and vomiting, and photophobia or phonophobia can be present, but not both. Interestingly, muscle tension or pain is not considered to be a fundamental component of diagnosis.

What are the symptoms of chronic daily headache?

Chronic daily headache is a descriptive term rather than a formal diagnostic term. It denotes frequent headache patterns of >15 days per month with at least 4 hours of headache during each of these days. Typically, there is a low-grade near-daily headache with episodes of severe, more migraine-like headaches superimposed. Consequently, a spectrum of symptoms can accompany this condition. The evolution of this headache pattern has been called transformation, suggesting that biological factors and time may be predisposing factors. This headache pattern can be maintained by overuse of analgesics. At other times, head and neck trauma may be an antecedent.

How will I know if I have a brain tumour?

Brain tumours are uncommon events and headache is rare as the only manifestation of a brain tumour. Typically, brain tumours present other neurological symptoms associated with a headache. The headache is of relatively recent onset (weeks to months) and progressive in nature. The remote risk of brain tumours and other secondary pathology underscores the value in establishing an ongoing relationship with the headache patient.

Is there a cure for migraine?

There is no cure for migraine, but it can be managed effectively in almost all instances. Migraine reflects the way the nervous system works. Attacks of migraine occur when the nervous system is disrupted by a migraine-provoking environment. Thus, adjusting lifestyle, understanding how the nervous system works and establishing a partnership with the medical provider are paramount for success. Successful people who have migraine are found in all walks of life.

What can be done to prevent migraine?

The foundation for preventing migraine is understanding the relationship of the nervous system with its environment. Learning to avoid or modify factors likely to provoke migraine and creating positive coping and lifestyle strategies to balance stress are the ultimate goals. There are a wide range of pharmacological measures that provide valuable support if needed. Alternative therapies, though not as thoroughly studied, may also be useful. Non-pharmacological strategies such as biofeedback, stress reduction techniques or cognitive restructuring can also prevent migraine.

Can a pharmacist treat migraine?

Pharmacists are key members of the support system for those with migraine. They are knowledgeable about prescription and non-prescription medications and a source for education about treatment of migraine. Many also provide vital links to screening. Working with a specific pharmacist who knows the medications and remedies you are taking can prevent many medication problems. Instructions are also available on the optimal use of medications, possible side-effects and benefits. Pharmacists do not formally diagnose disease but have enough general knowledge to provide considerable guidance about migraine care.

Do I need to see a doctor about migraine?

Some people with mild or infrequent migraine can self-manage their disease without medical supervision. However, many people who self-manage their disease are not achieving quality outcomes. Delaying evaluation can lead to considerable lost time and disruption of personal and family life. If you have recurrent headaches that interfere with your ability to function despite your best efforts to treat, you should consult your physician. Furthermore, medical consultation should be considered if you are using any treatment more than three times a month. Today, more than ever, migraine is a treatable disease. The cornerstone of successful treatment is an accurate diagnosis and a personalized management plan. The use of prescription medications helps most sufferers. Therefore, physicians are key members of the migraine support system.

Do I need drugs every day to prevent migraine?

Most people with migraine do not need preventative medications. However, if migraines are frequent or difficult to treat, preventative medications can be invaluable. The purpose of preventative medications is to provide support to your nervous system so that it can effectively resist migraines. In most instances, many different factors put the nervous system at risk for migraine and, consequently, preventative medications need to be taken daily. Sometimes, when there is a predictable time or risk factor, such as the menses, a preventative medication may be taken only around that event. In most instances, medications only need to be used for a limited period of time. Lifestyle adjustments or establishing strategies to modify risk factors can be valuable adjuncts and often limit the need for preventative medications.

Preventative medications may also be used if no acute treatment has proved effective, or if the patient wishes to use therapies on a regular basis to prevent their migraine.

What drugs will I need for my migraine?

Almost all people use some kind of medication to treat their attacks of migraine, but the medication is less than effective for nearly half of them. The range of medications available varies considerably. Common medications include a variety of prescription and over-the-counter pain medications, prescription medications for nausea and prescription medications for migraine, which are the most effective therapies. Prescription medications may be in the form of tablets, nasal sprays or injections. Many patients use more than one type of medication or combinations of these products to treat the various presentations of migraine they experience. The most important attribute of a medication for treating migraine is that it safely and consistently aborts the migraine. In addition, there are prescription medications and herbal remedies that may prevent migraine when taken on a regular basis.

What are triptans?

Triptans are a class of medications that are designed specifically to treat attacks of migraine. They are chemically designed to mimic serotonin, a chemical used by nerves to communicate with each other. Serotonin levels are low during migraine and triptan drugs assist the nervous system with re-establishing control of function. There are several triptans that are currently available and, although they differ slightly in their chemical characteristics, they all function in the same manner.

How do triptans work?

Migraine is a complex process that can affect the body in many ways. During migraine attacks, blood vessels around the brain can swell and become inflamed. As this happens, the nervous system's ability to block pain is decreased. Triptans work by decreasing the swelling and inflammation of the blood vessels involved in the migraine process. They also restore the nervous system's ability to block pain impulses. This is why they are considered migraine-specific medications.

Is it safe to take triptans?

Triptans are one of the most thoroughly studied drugs ever. They have been used by millions of migraine sufferers and for literally hundreds of millions of migraine attacks. They have an excellent overall safety profile. However, as with all medications, they are not perfect. There have been rare reports of cardiac problems associated with triptan use. It is therefore important to discuss your risk for heart disease with your medical provider. In addition, there are certain medications that should not be taken with a triptan and there are specific types of headache for which a triptan should not be given. These issues too should be discussed with your medical provider.

When is the best time to take my migraine medications?

For most people with migraine, taking medication early in the attack gives the best results. Not only do the medications work better, but also the time the migraine interferes with your life is reduced considerably. Most drugs, e.g. analgesics and ergotamine, should be taken as early as possible, during the prodrome or aura phases if possible. Triptans should be delayed till the headache is mild, but not left till it is moderate or severe. Triptans are not only more effective when taken during mild headaches, but the migraine is also less likely to recur. For many sufferers this can result in using less medication. However, an early treatment strategy may not be advised for those with very frequent migraines or those who cannot predict that the mild headache will advance to a more severe headache. Diaries can be very helpful in monitoring treatment response.

Can I try acupuncture and herbal remedies for migraine?

Even though there have been few scientific studies to address the usefulness of acupuncture and herbal remedies for migraine, mainly due to the cost of such research, the best judge to measure the outcome of these treatment modalities is you. To date, small studies of these treatments have been somewhat equivocal. However, from a practical standpoint, the real question is: can these treatments help you? From that perspective, you and your provider can try these modalities and monitor them for benefit. This is best done with a diary and establishing objective criteria for success.

What is the best way to treat tension-type headache?

Treatment for tension-type headache is best determined by the circumstances that accompany the headache. If tension-type headache is isolated and the only type of headache a person experiences, it may be treated with rest, sleep, exercise or possibly a simple non-prescription analgesic. If tension headaches are frequent, then preventative medications are recommended. If tension headache is often a harbinger to migraine then it should be treated as such. If tension headache is a component of chronic daily headache, then treatment needs to be comprehensive.

I get headaches every day. What can I do?

Daily headaches present a challenge for medical providers and patients alike. Having daily headaches suggests that the nervous system itself is sensitized and its pain-suppressing abilities impaired. Many factors may be associated with the development of chronic daily headaches. Probably the most important, because it is reversible, is the overuse of medications used to treat attacks of migraine. Whenever daily headaches are associated with daily use of treatment medication, then that medication itself may be perpetuating the headache. Typical of this condition is a history of episodic headache in earlier life that over time evolves into a daily headache pattern. Once established, the offending medication may temporarily relieve the headache, but as the medicine is excreted, the headache returns, requiring more medication, which continues the cycle. Medicines that are commonly associated with this condition are opioid analgesics (e.g. codeine), ergotamines, butalbital products and caffeine-containing products. The key to managing this condition is to discontinue the use of the offending medication. This generally requires medical assistance. Head trauma and genetic factors may also be associated with daily headaches. Some headache experts believe that poorly controlled headaches expedite the evolution of episodic headaches into chronic daily headaches.

Antibiotics don't work for my sinus headaches. What can I do?

Many people commonly experience head and facial pain localized to the sinus area. Infrequently, this can be part of an infectious process called sinusitis. In these instances antibiotics are typically prescribed. However, far more often, recurrent episodes of pain in this area associated with nasal congestion or even tearing of the eyes are migraines. Ironically, migraine is a far more frequent cause of these symptoms than is infection. These symptoms occur during migraine because the same nerve that goes to blood vessels around the brain also goes into the sinus area. If branches of that nerve are activated during migraine then nasal symptoms are noted. It is therefore important to be given an accurate diagnosis.

How can I control my migraines?
The most successful way to control migraines is to establish a management partnership with your healthcare provider. Be willing to assume an active decision-making role, seek out information and develop a curiosity about your own nervous system. Investigate factors that may provoke or prevent migraine, learn your body's "early warning system" that communicates when the nervous system is distressed, and treat migraine attacks effectively with clear goals of success in mind. The best tool for accomplishing long-term migraine control is a headache calendar/diary.

Future Developments in Migraine Management

There are currently several ongoing initiatives to improve migraine diagnosis and management in the clinic, including:

- Evidence-based guidelines for headache management in primary care.
- Impact-based recognition of migraine.
- Phase-specific treatment of migraine.
- New migraine therapies in development.

These initiatives are in varying stages of development and implementation, and should be introduced into specialist and general clinical practice over the next few years.

Evidence-based guidelines for headache management in primary care

Primary care is unique among medical specialties and requires its own set of management tools. For example, primary care practitioners work under greater demands to evaluate more patients in a shorter time span than most specialists. In the context of primary care, practitioners frequently are prioritizing many divergent patient complaints and at the same time attempting to integrate preventative and health maintenance efforts. Thus, primary care providers need tools that are time efficient and directed to appropriate decisions of care.

When patients are referred to a consultant, they are most often presenting with specific disease complaints. Most efforts to provide clinical guidelines are created by specialists and are pathology-based, with a focus on a specific disease state. In this context, clinical guidelines created by specialists are more appropriate for their own method of practice.

Patients entering the medical system at the primary care level often bring multiple concerns and diverse undifferentiated symptomatology. Physicians are required to manage patients, not just specific disease entities. Consequently, guidelines are needed that focus on patient management and the early evolution of disease conditions. They need to focus on early recognition of diseases for which treatment is available and provide clear outcome expectations for patients. As principles of care, guidelines should be instruments to prioritize patients quickly into appropriate management algorithms.

Impact-based recognition of migraine

Traditionally, the diagnosis of migraine has been symptom-based. However, the symptoms of various primary headache disorders are not symptomatically distinct and specific symptoms do not necessarily create diagnostic exclusivity. In fact, there is considerable overlap in the symptoms that diagnostically differentiate migraine from migrainous headache, tension-type headache or even so-called "sinus" headache. Symptoms differentiating the nuances of these various headache diagnoses are, to a significant degree, an academic exercise, since treatment paradigms overlap and most patients meet diagnostic criteria for multiple headache diagnoses. While these diagnostic nuances appear to have considerable significance for medical academia, in the pragmatic world of primary care the distinctions are often a source of confusion and indifference. Recent research has demonstrated that patients with only episodic tension-type headache are rare in clinical practice[31] and that most patients believe they have multiple headache types, regardless of medical diagnosis. From the perspective of patient care, the ability to successfully manage patients is more critical than finding the correct academic diagnosis.

Compounding these issues is the fact that current symptom-based diagnostic criteria were developed for clinical research trials. They answer the question of when a specific headache is unquestionably a migraine. In clinical trials, the symptoms of migraine, unhindered by treatment efforts, progressed until the headache and associated symptoms were fully developed. This resulted in prolongation of the disability and decreased the likelihood of complete response, at least for the oral triptans. In clinical practice, patients frequently describe their headache symptoms coincident with efforts to treat. These interventions may distort or eliminate some key diagnostic symptoms and thus obscure the diagnosis.

In primary care practice, the diagnostic and therapeutic goals are quite different. Diagnostically, the question is how soon can a disabling migraine be identified and intervention begin to shorten or eliminate the disabling impact of the migraine. This distinction has led to the development of a migraine recognition scheme based on the historical pattern of headache impact rather than specific symptom constellations. Consequently, in this scheme, migraine is defined as a stable pattern of recurrent disabling headache.

The rationale for an impact-based recognition scheme is that the medical relevance of migraine is largely related to the degree of disruption migraine produces for a given individual. This in turn is the major determinant of treatment need. In the Spectrum Study, it was demonstrated that within populations of patients diagnosed by IHS criteria as having migraine and significant headache-related disability, their entire spectrum of primary headaches responded equally well to oral sumatriptan.[78] Furthermore, a similar treatment response was reported in a smaller population of subjects with diagnosed disabling migrainous headache. This population did not have a history of "true" migraine. Finally, subjects diagnosed with only episodic tension-type headache and having significant headache-related disability were uncommon in clinical practice.[31] Thus, headaches associated with significant disability are very likely to be migraine and responsive to triptans.

The impact-based recognition scheme consists of four questions:

- Do your headaches interfere with your ability to work or engage in family and social functions?
- Has the pattern of your headache changed over the last 6 months?
- How frequently do you have any kind of headaches?
- What are you doing to treat your headaches?[5]

The first question quickly separates medically relevant headaches from those more trivial in nature. Migraine should be considered the default diagnosis for headache that significantly interferes with a person's ability to function. Probing for examples of how function is disrupted allows the provider to assess treatment needs and creates rapport with the patient. A positive response necessitates query for migraine-specific associations such as the presence of nausea, sensory sensitivity, positive family history and, in women, menstrual association.

The second question is designed to alert the provider to sinister headache conditions. A new or different headache mandates a thorough diagnostic approach, while a stable headache pattern provides reassurance to the provider and patient.

The third question alerts the provider to chronic headache patterns. In turn, this relates to consideration of prophylactic medications and tempers the use of acute treatment medications.

The fourth question screens for medication overuse and the effectiveness of self-treatment efforts.

Impact-based recognition is a time-efficient screening method that allows providers to quickly screen patients for headache in the out-patient setting, even when they are being evaluated for other complaints.

Phase-specific treatment of migraine

Migraine results from a neurological process that evolves through several phases over time (see pp. 10–16).[4] Headache is one of many symptoms that can evolve out of this process. The process of migraine can be conceptualized into pre-headache, headache and post-headache phases. Therapeutic interventions can be based on the different phases of migraine (Figure 46).[5]

Treatment during the prodrome

The efficacy of many therapeutic interventions is significantly dependent on the phase of migraine in which treatment is initiated. This is particularly true for the triptan drugs. During the premonitory period, simply removing oneself from stressful environments or engaging in relaxation or biofeedback can often abort the impending migraine. Some preliminary studies

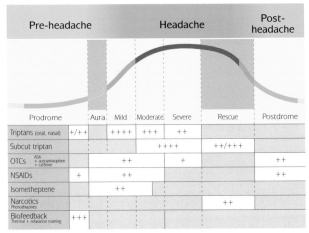

Figure 46. Phase-specific acute therapy for migraine. Reprinted with permission from reference 5; copyright Primary Care Network, 2000.

indicate that acute treatments may be effective when taken during the prodrome. One small study demonstrated that naratriptan reduced or eliminated almost 80% of predicted headaches when taken during the premonitory period.[90] Similar older studies of DHE have demonstrated the same results.[68] NSAIDs have also been suggested for use in this role.

Treatment during the migraine aura
Many pharmacological therapies have been suggested to treat aura, but none has clear evidence of efficacy. For example, there is little evidence for the efficacy of triptans when taken during the aura period.[171,172] However, if simple auras are consistently followed by headache, treatment with oral preparations can be initiated to prevent the unnecessary delay of waiting for the headache. However, this strategy is not recommended for complex aura symptomatology.

Treatment during the mild headache phase
Many headache specialists have encouraged treating headache early. However, with the advent of triptans and the clinical

trial methodology requiring headaches to be not treated until they were moderate to severe,[60] therapeutic benefits for early intervention with triptans were not appreciated. Recent analysis of protocol violators who treated some migraines when the headache was mild suggested the efficacy was dramatically improved over efficacy when treating moderate to severe headache.[58]

More recently, a prospective, randomized, placebo-controlled study has supported these observations.[70] In addition, there appears to be less recurrence of headache and the time to resolution of migraine is diminished.[173] This strongly suggests that, for properly selected patients, initiating triptans during the mild phase of headache reduces the overall impact of an attack of migraine.

Selecting patients appropriate for this strategy is important. Ideally, there should be a high correlation between the onset of mild headache and its evolution to moderate to severe headache. This is not a recommended strategy for patients with very frequent headache attacks since it could lead to analgesic overuse.

Treatment during moderate to severe headache

Most of the evidence from clinical trials is derived from pharmacological interventions during the moderate to severe headache phase of migraine. A wide range of drugs have reported efficacy for relieving pain and associated migraine symptoms. The most effective are the triptans, but analgesics and anti-emetics also have utility (see section on "Headache Treatments").

Treatment using rescue medication

Occasionally an attack of migraine may not respond to initial therapeutic interventions. In order to prevent unnecessary utilization of healthcare resources and provide relief, it is often wise to provide patients with a rescue therapy in advance. Commonly used products are subcutaneous sumatriptan, butorphanol nasal spray (*not available in Europe*) and parenteral phenothiazines. It is important to monitor the frequency of use of rescue therapies. In general, if patients require rescue more than once or twice a month, then first-line acute therapy should be adjusted, efforts to initiate interventions earlier in the migraine process encouraged and/or the addition of prophylactic medications instituted. In addition, coping stategies and resources of the patient should be assessed.

Treatment during the post-headache phase

Many patients report that they experience significant impact from migraine in the post-headache period. Little formal study has been given to this phase of migraine but, in general, simple analgesics and NSAIDs improve symptoms. Re-hydration is also recommended.

Phase-specific treatment can be an effective strategy for many patients with migraine. It encourages their vigilance and participation in treatment. It also affords the opportunity to intervene early and with specific efforts. This, in many patients, limits the impact of migraine and reduces treatment failures.

New migraine therapies in development

As well as the several new triptans in various stages of development, the co-administration of triptans with other medications is being investigated:

- The combination of a triptan with an analgesic (e.g. an NSAID), with or without an anti-emetic to improve gastric motility, has the potential to provide synergistic effects on migraine pain and associated symptoms over and above that provided by the triptan alone.
- The co-administration of a long half-life triptan (e.g. naratriptan) together with a faster-acting triptan (e.g. sumatriptan) has potential for the treatment of patients who frequently report headache recurrence following triptan therapy.

New prophylactic medications are also being developed, including botulinum toxin and tizanidine.

Botulinum toxin

Botulinum toxin is elaborated by *Clostridium botulinum* and multiple serotypes are known to exist. Serotypes A and B

(Botox and Myoblock, respectively) are in the initial phases of study for migraine prevention. A double-blind, placebo-controlled study has demonstrated that botulinum A (Botox) has the potential to reduce the frequency and severity of migraine attacks.[174] However, controlled studies with Botox in tension-type headache have yielded equivocal results.[175–177]

Tizanidine

Tizanidine is an alpha-2-adrenergic agonist that is indicated for spasticity associated with multiple sclerosis and other diseases. It is currently in clinical development by Athena Neurosciences for the prophylaxis of headaches. Small open studies have indicated that tizanidine has promise for the prophylaxis of chronic daily headache,[178] migraine,[179] chronic tension-type headache[180] and in the detoxification from analgesic rebound headache.[181]

To the future

The disease of migraine has undergone an amazing transition in the last decade. This is in large part the result of research into the basic science of migraine. From these efforts, acute treatments such as the triptans were developed, which revolutionized migraine management. More recently, advancement has been witnessed in the clinical science of migraine as well. Today, migraine is probably the most successfully managed neurological disease.

Clearly, much more work lies ahead. While acute therapies have arrived at a frenzied pace, preventative therapies have not. Understanding the spectrum and longitudinal history of migraine as it relates to other headache disorders, co-morbidities and chronic daily headache is an obvious clinical need. There is much yet to accomplish. However, it is important to keep in mind that primary care provides the foundation and platform from which headache care will advance clinically. While there is much to do, there is today much to offer those suffering from migraine.

References

1. Headache Classification Committee of the International Headache Society. Classification and diagnostic criteria for headache disorders, cranial neuralgias and facial pain. *Cephalalgia* 1988; **8**(Suppl 7): 19–28.

2. Breslau N, Rasmussen BK. The impact of migraine: epidemiology, risk factors, and co-morbidities. *Neurology* 2001; **56**(Suppl 1): 4–12.

3. Stewart WF, Lipton RB, Celentano DD *et al*. Prevalence of migraine headache in the United States. Relation to age, income, race and other sociodemographic factors. *J Am Med Assoc* 1992; **267**: 64–69.

4. Blau JN, Drummond MF. *Migraine*. London: Office of Health Economics, 1991.

5. Bedell AW, Cady RK, Diamond ML *et al*. *Patient-centered Strategies for Effective Management of Migraine*. Primary Care Network, 2000.

6. Blau JN. The clinical diagnosis of migraine: the beginning of therapy. *J Neurol* 1991; **238**: S6–S11.

7. Micieli G. Suffering in silence. In: Edmeads J, editor. *Migraine: A Brighter Future*. Worthing: Cambridge Medical Publications, 1993; pp. 1–7.

8. Stewart WF, Shechter A, Lipton RB. Migraine heterogeneity. Disability, pain intensity, and attack frequency and duration. *Neurology* 1994; **44**(Suppl 4): 24–39.

9. National Academy of Sciences/Institute of Medicine (NAS/IOM). *Disability in America: Toward a National Agenda for Prevention*. Washington, DC: NAS Press, 1991.

10. Clarke CE, MacMillan L, Sondhi S *et al*. Economic and social impact of migraine. *Q J Med* 1996; **89**: 77–84.

11. Dowson A, Jagger S. The UK migraine patient survey: quality of life and treatment. *Curr Med Res Opin* 1999; **15**: 241–253.

12. Von Korff M, Stewart WF, Simon DJ *et al*. Migraine and reduced work performance: a population-based diary study. *Neurology* 1998; **50**: 1741–1745.

13. Von Korff M, Ormel J, Keefe FJ *et al*. Grading the severity of chronic pain. *Pain* 1992; **50**: 133–149.

14. Abu-Arefeh I, Russell G. Prevalence of headache and migraine in schoolchildren. *Br Med J* 1994; **309**: 765–769.

15. Ferrari MD. The economic burden of migraine to society. *Pharmacoeconomics* 1998; **13**: 667–676.

16. Smith RC. Impact of migraine on the family. *Headache* 1996; **36**: 278 (Abstract).

17. Kryst S, Scherl ER. Social and personal impact of headache in Kentucky. In: Olesen J, editor. *Headache Classification and Epidemiology*. New York: Raven Press, 1994; pp. 345–350.

18. Osterhaus JT, Townsend RJ, Gandek B *et al*. Measuring the functional status and well-being of patients with migraine headache. *Headache* 1994; **34**: 337–343.

19. Dahlöf CGH, Dimenas E. Migraine patients experience poorer subjective well-being/quality of life even between attacks. *Cephalalgia* 1995; **15**: 31–36.

20. Blau JN. Fears aroused in patients by migraine. *Br Med J* 1984; **288**: 1126.

21. Liddell J. Migraine: the patient's perspective. *Rev Contemp Pharmacother* 1994; **5**: 253–257.

22. Russell MB, Olesen J. Increased familial risk and evidence of genetic factors in migraine. *Br Med J* 1995; **311**: 541–544.

23. Mathew NT. Pathophysiology, epidemiology, and impact of migraine. *Clin Cornerstone* 2001; **4**: 1–17.

24. Goadsby PJ, Olesen J. Diagnosis and management of migraine. *Br Med J* 1996; **312**: 1279–1283.

25. Weiller C, May A, Limmroth V *et al*. Brain stem activation in spontaneous human migraine attacks. *Nature Med* 1995; **1**: 658–660.

26. Staffa JA, Lipton RB, Stewart WF. The epidemiology of migraine headache. *Rev Contemp Pharmacother* 1994; **5**: 241–252.

27. Peatfield RC, Olesen J. Migraine: precipitating factors. In: Olesen J, Tfelt-Hansen P, Welch KMA, editors. *The Headaches*. New York: Raven Press, 1993; pp. 241–245.

28. Silberstein SD, Lipton RB. Chronic daily headache. *Curr Opin Neurol* 2000; **13**: 277–283.

29. Olesen J. Analgesic headache. A common, treatable condition that deserves more attention. *Br Med J* 1995; **310**: 479–480.

30. Couch JR, Bearss C. Chronic daily headache in the post-trauma syndrome: relation to extent of head injury. *Headache* 2001; **41**: 559–564.

31. Lipton RB, Cady RK, Stewart WF *et al.* Diagnostic lessons from the Spectrum study. *Neurology* 2002; in press.

32. Dowson AJ, Gruffydd-Jones K, Hackett G *et al. Migraine: Key Facts. Essential Information from MIPCA*. Richmond: Synergy Medical Education, 1998.

33. Silberstein SD, Lipton RB, Goadsby PJ. *Headache in Clinical Practice*. Oxford: Isis Medical Media, 1998.

34. Bird N, MacGregor EA, Wilkinson MI. Ice cream headache – site, duration, and relationship to migraine. *Headache* 1992; **32**: 35–38.

35. Matharu M, Goadsby PJ. Cluster headache: update on a common neurological problem. *Pract Neurol* 2001; **1**: 42–49.

36. Kost RG, Straus SE. Post-herpetic neuralgia – pathogenesis, treatment and prevention. *New Engl J Med* 1996; **335**: 32–42.

37. Cawson RA. Temporomandibular cephalagia. In: Clifford Rose F, editor. *Handbook of Clinical Neurology*. Amsterdam: Elsevier, 1986; Vol. 4, pp. 413–416.

38. Lipton RB, Stewart WF, Liberman J *et al*. Patterns of healthcare utilization for migraine in England. *Cephalalgia* 1999; **19**: 305 (Abstract).

39. Edmeads J, Findlay H, Tugwell P *et al*. Impact of migraine and tension-type headache on life-style, consulting behaviour, and medication use: a Canadian population survey. *Can J Neurol Sci* 1993; **20**: 131–137.

40. Lipton RB, Stewart WF, Simon D. Medical consultation for migraine: results from the American Migraine Study. *Headache* 1998; **38**: 87–96.

41. Rasmussen BK, Jensen R, Olesen J. Impact of headache on sickness absence and utilisation of medical services: a Danish population study. *J Epidemiol Community Health* 1992; **46**: 443–446.

42. Sakai F, Igarashi H. Epidemiology of migraine in Japan. *Cephalalgia* 1997; **17**: 15–22.

43. Stang PE, Osterhaus JT, Celentano DD. Migraine. Patterns of healthcare use. *Neurology* 1994; **44**(Suppl 4): 47–55.

44. Stang PE, Von Korff M. The diagnosis of headache in primary care: factors in the agreement of clinical and standardized diagnoses. *Headache* 1994; **34**: 138–142.

45. Richard A, Massiou H, Herrmann MA. Frequency and profile of migraine patients seen by general practitioners. *Semin Hosp Paris* 1999; **75**: 440–446.

46. Holmes W, Laughey W, MacGregor EA *et al*. Headache consultation and referral patterns in one UK general practice. *Cephalalgia* 1999; **19**: 328–329 (Abstract).

47. MacGregor EA. An international study assessing the impact of migraine on the behavioural and social activities of sufferers who consult pharmacists. *Proc 59th Int Cong FIP* 1999; 128 (Abstract).

48. Celentano DD, Stewart WF, Lipton RB *et al*. Medication use and disability among migraineurs: a national probability sample survey. *Headache* 1992; **32**: 223–228.

49. Lipton RB, Stewart WF. Acute migraine therapy: do doctors understand what patients want from therapy? *Headache* 1999; **39**(Suppl 2): 20–26.

50. Edmeads J, Láinez JM, Brandes JL *et al*. Potential of the Migraine Disability Assessment (MIDAS) Questionnaire as a public health initiative and in clinical practice. *Neurology* 2001; **56**(Suppl 1): S29–S34.

51. Steiner TJ, MacGregor EA, Davies PTG. Guidelines for all doctors in the diagnosis and management of migraine and tension-type headache. British Association for the Study of Headache, 2000; www.bash.org.uk

52. Lewis TA, Solomon GD. Advances in migraine management. *Cleveland Clin J Med* 1995; **62**: 148–155.

53. Diener HC, Brune K, Gerber WD *et al*. Therapy of acute migraine attacks and migraine prophylaxis – guidelines of the German Migraine and Headache Society [in German]. *Nervenheilkunde* 1997; **16**: 500–510.

54. Dowson AJ, Gruffydd-Jones K, Hackett G *et al*. *Migraine Management Guidelines*. London: Synergy Medical Education, 2000.

55. Matchar DB, Young WB, Rosenberg JH *et al*. Multispecialty consensus on diagnosis and treatment of headache: pharmacological management of acute attacks. *Neurology* 2000; **54**(8): 1553. www.aan.com/public/practiceguidelines/03.pdf

56. Lipton RB, Silberstein SD. The role of headache-related disability in migraine management. *Neurology* 2001; **56**(Suppl 1): S35–S42.

57. Lipton RB. Disability assessment as a basis for stratified care. *Cephalalgia* 1998; **18**(Suppl 22): 40–46.

58. Cady RK, Sheftell F, Lipton RB *et al*. Early treatment with sumatriptan enhances pain-free response: retrospective analysis from three clinical trials. *Clin Ther* 2000; **22**: 1035–1048.

59. Ramadan NM, Silberstein SD, Freitag FG *et al*. Multispecialty consensus on diagnosis and treatment of headache: pharmacological management for prevention of migraine. *Neurology* 2000; **54**(8): 1553. www.aan.com/public/practiceguidelines/05.pdf

60. Pilgrim AJ. Methodology of clinical trials of sumatriptan in migraine and cluster headache. *Eur Neurol* 1991; **31**: 295–299.

61. Lanza FL. Endoscopic studies of gastric and duodenal injury after the use of ibuprofen, aspirin, and other nonsteroidal anti-inflammatory agents. *Am J Med* 1984; **77**: 19–24.

62. Dowson A, Ball K, Haworth D. Comparison of a fixed combination of domperidone and paracetamol (Domperamol) with sumatriptan 50 mg in moderate to severe migraine: a randomised UK primary care study. *Curr Med Res Opin* 2000; **16**: 190–197.

63. Freitag FG, Cady R, DiSerio F *et al*. Comparative study of a combination of isometheptene mucate, dichloralphenazone with acetaminophen and sumatriptan succinate in the treatment of migraine. *Headache* 2001; **41**: 391–398.

64. Olesen J. A review of current drugs for migraine. *J Neurol* 1991; **238**: S23–S27.

65. Winner P, Ricalde O, Leforce B *et al*. A double-blind study of subcutaneous dihydroergotamine vs. subcutaneous sumatriptan in the treatment of acute migraine. *Arch Neurol* 1996; **53**: 180–184.

66. Touchon J, Bertin L, Pilgrim AJ *et al*. A comparison of subcutaneous sumatriptan and dihydroergotamine nasal spray in the acute treatment of migraine. *Neurology* 1996; **47**: 361–365.

67. Boureau F, Kappos L, Schoenen J *et al*. A clinical comparison of sumatriptan nasal spray and dihydroergotamine nasal spray in the acute treatment of migraine. *Int J Clin Pract* 2000; **54**: 281–286.

68. Massiou H. Dihydroergotamine nasal spray in prevention and treatment of migraine attacks: two controlled trials versus placebo. *Cephalalgia* 1987; **7**(Suppl 6): 440–441.

69. Connor HE, Beattie DT. 5-Hydroxytryptamine receptor subtypes and migraine. In: Sandler M, Ferrari M, Harnett S, editors. *Migraine: Pharmacology and Genetics*. London: Chapman & Hall, 1996; pp. 18–31.

70. Cady RK, Lipton RB, Hall C *et al*. Treatment of mild headache in disabled migraine sufferers: results of the Spectrum study. *Headache* 2000; **40**: 792–797.

71. Welch KM, Mathew NT, Stone P *et al*. Tolerability of sumatriptan: clinical trials and post-marketing experience. *Cephalalgia* 2000; **20**: 687–695.

72. Sheftell FD, Fox AW. Acute migraine treatment outcome measures: a clinician's view. *Cephalalgia* 2000; **20**(Suppl 2): 14–24.

73. Pfaffenrath V, Cunin G, Sjonell G *et al*. Efficacy and safety of sumatriptan tablets (25 mg, 50 mg, and 100 mg) in the acute treatment of migraine: defining the optimum doses of oral sumatriptan. *Headache* 1998; **38**: 184–190.

74. Multinational Oral Sumatriptan and Cafergot Comparative Study Group. A randomized, double-blind comparison of sumatriptan and Cafergot in the acute treatment of migraine. *Eur Neurol* 1991; **31**: 314–322.

75. Oral Sumatriptan and Aspirin-plus-Metoclopramide Comparative Study Group. A study to compare oral sumatriptan with oral aspirin plus oral metoclopramide in the acute treatment of migraine. *Eur Neurol* 1992; **32**: 177–184.

76. Tfelt-Hansen P, Henry P, Mulder LJ *et al.* The effectiveness of combined oral lysine acetylsalicylate and metoclopramide compared with oral sumatriptan for migraine. *Lancet* 1995; **346**: 923–926.

77. Myllylä VV, Havanka H, Herrala L *et al.* Tolfenamic acid rapid release versus sumatriptan in the acute treatment of migraine: comparable effect in a double-blind, randomized, controlled, parallel-group study. *Headache* 1998; **38**: 201–207.

78. Lipton RB, Stewart WF, Cady RK *et al.* Sumatriptan for the range of headaches in migraine sufferers: results of the Spectrum Study. *Headache* 2000; **40**: 783–791.

79. Salonen R, Ashford E, Dahlöf C *et al.*, for the International Intranasal Sumatriptan Study Group. Intranasal sumatriptan for the acute treatment of migraine. *J Neurol* 1994; **241**: 463–469.

80. Ryan R, Elkind A, Baker CC *et al.* Sumatriptan nasal spray for the acute treatment of migraine. Results of two clinical studies. *Neurology* 1997; **49**: 1225–1230.

81. Rothner AD, Winner P, Nett R *et al.* One-year tolerability and efficacy of sumatriptan nasal spray in adolescents with migraine: results of a multicenter, open-label study. *Clin Ther* 2000; **22**: 1533–1546.

82. Hershey AD, Powers SW, LeCates S *et al.* Effectiveness of nasal sumatriptan in 5- to 12-year-old children. *Headache* 2001; **41**: 693–697.

83. Carpay HA, Matthijsse P, Steinbuch M *et al.* Oral and subcutaneous sumatriptan in the acute treatment of migraine: an open randomized cross-over study. *Cephalalgia* 1997; **17**: 591–595.

84. Gruffydd-Jones K, Hood CA, Price DB. A within-patient comparison of subcutaneous and oral sumatriptan in the acute treatment of migraine in general practice. *Cephalalgia* 1997; **17**: 31–36.

85. Klassen A, Elkind A, Asgharnejad M *et al.* Naratriptan is effective and well tolerated in the acute treatment of migraine. Results of a double-blind, placebo-controlled, parallel-group study. *Headache* 1997; **37**: 640–645.

86. Mathew NT, Asgharnejad M, Peykamian M *et al.* Naratriptan is effective and well tolerated in the acute treatment of migraine. Results of a double-blind, placebo-controlled, crossover study. *Neurology* 1997; **49**: 1485–1490.

87. Salonen R. Naratriptan. *Int J Clin Pract* 1999; **53**: 552–556.

88. Sheftell FD, Rapoport AM, Coddon DR. Naratriptan in the prophylaxis of transformed migraine. *Headache* 1999; **39**: 506–510.

89. Newman L, Mannix LK, Landy S *et al*. Naratriptan as short-term prophylaxis of menstrually associated migraine: a randomized, double-blind, placebo-controlled study. *Headache* 2001; **41**: 248–256.

90. Luciani R, Carter D, Mannix L *et al*. Prevention of migraine during prodrome with naratriptan. *Cephalalgia* 2000; **20**: 122–126.

91. Eekers PJ, Koehler PJ. Naratriptan prophylactic treatment in cluster headache. *Cephalalgia* 2001; **21**: 75–76.

92. Silberstein S. Zolmitriptan is effective in the treatment of menstrually associated migraine attacks. *Cephalalgia* 2001; **21**: 420 (Abstract).

93. Linder SL, Dowson AJ. Zolmitriptan provides effective migraine relief in adolescents. *Int J Clin Pract* 2000; **54**: 466–469.

94. Dowson A, MacGregor EA, Brandes J *et al*. Zolmitriptan orally disintegrating tablets provide effective, convenient migraine relief. *Cephalalgia* 2001; **21**: 419–420 (Abstract).

95. Purdy A, Reunanen M, Lee D. High efficacy and tolerability nasal spray extends to long-term treatment of migraine. *Cephalalgia* 2001; **21**: 418–419 (Abstract).

96. Pascual J, Peris F, Cabarrocas X *et al*. Meta-analysis of the efficacy of almotriptan for the treatment of acute migraine attacks. *Cephalalgia* 2001; **21**: 427 (Abstract).

97. Dodick DW. Oral almotriptan in the treatment of migraine: safety and tolerability. *Headache* 2001; **41**: 449–455.

98. Diener HC, McHarg A. Pharmacology and efficacy of eletriptan for the treatment of migraine attacks. *Int J Clin Pract* 2000; **54**: 670–674.

99. Goadsby PJ, Ferrari MD, Olesen J *et al*. Eletriptan in acute migraine: a double-blind, placebo-controlled comparison to sumatriptan. *Neurology* 2000; **54**: 156–163.

100. Easthope CE, Goa KL. Frovatriptan. *CNS Drugs* 2001; **15**: 969–976.

101. Ryan R, Keywood C. Frovatriptan: review of efficacy in acute treatment of migraine. In: *Montreal 2000. Proceedings of the 42nd Annual Scientific Meeting of the American Headache Society, 2000*: p. 230 (Abstract).

102. Goebel H, Winter P, Boswell D *et al*. Comparison of naratriptan and sumatriptan in recurrence-prone migraine patients. *Clin Ther* 2000; **22**: 981–989.

103. Havanka H, Dahlöf C, Pop PH *et al*. Efficacy of naratriptan tablets in the acute treatment of migraine: a dose-ranging study. *Clin Ther* 2000; **22**: 970–980.

104. Stark S, Spierings EL, McNeal S *et al*. Naratriptan efficacy in migraineurs who respond poorly to oral sumatriptan. *Headache* 2000; **40**: 513–520.

105. Gruffydd-Jones K, Kies B, Middleton A *et al*. Zolmitriptan versus sumatriptan for the acute oral treatment of migraine: a randomized, double-blind, international study. *Eur J Neurol* 2001; **8**: 237–245.

106. Pascual J, Munoz R, Leira R. An open preference study with sumatriptan 50 mg and zolmitriptan 2.5 mg in 100 migraine patients. *Cephalalgia* 2001; **21**: 680–684.

107. Adelman JU, Lipton RB, Ferrari MD *et al*. Comparison of rizatriptan and other triptans on stringent measures of efficacy. *Neurology* 2001; **57**: 1377–1383.

108. Gerth WC, McCarroll KA, Santanello NC *et al*. Patient satisfaction with rizatriptan versus other triptans: direct head-to-head comparisons. *Int J Clin Pract* 2001; **55**: 552–556.

109. Tfelt-Hansen P, Ryan RE Jr. Oral therapy for migraine: comparisons between rizatriptan and sumatriptan. A review of four randomized, double-blind clinical trials. *Neurology* 2000; **55**(9, Suppl 2): S19–S24.

110. Loder E, Brandes JL, Silberstein S *et al*. Preference comparison of rizatriptan ODT and sumatriptan 50 mg tablet in migraine. *Headache* 2001; **41**: 745–753.

111. Pascual J, Bussone G, Hernandez JF *et al*. Comparison of preference for rizatriptan 10 mg wafer versus sumatriptan 50 mg tablet in migraine. *Eur Neurol* 2001; **45**: 275–283.

112. Spierings EL, Gomez-Mancilla B, Grosz DE *et al*. Oral almotriptan vs. oral sumatriptan in the abortive treatment of migraine: a double-blind, randomized, parallel-group, optimum-dose comparison. *Arch Neurol* 2001; **58**: 944–950.

113. Fuseau E, Petricoul O, Sabin A *et al*. Effect of encapsulation on absorption of sumatriptan tablets: data from healthy volunteers and patients during a migraine. *Clin Ther* 2001; **23**: 242–251.

114. Ferrari MD, Roon KI, Lipton RB *et al*. Oral triptans (serotonin 5-HT$_{1B/1D}$ agonists) in acute migraine treatment: a meta-analysis of 53 trials. *Lancet* 2001; **358**: 1668–1675.

115. Diener HC, Limmroth V. The management of migraine. *Rev Contemp Pharmacother* 1994; **5**: 271–284.

116. Diener H-C, Föh M, Iaccarino C *et al*. Cyclandelate in the prophylaxis of migraine: a randomized, parallel, double-blind study in comparison with placebo and propranolol. *Cephalalgia* 1996; **16**: 441–447.

117. Ludin HP. Flunarizine and propranolol in the treatment of migraine. *Headache* 1989; **29**: 218–223.

118. Johnson RH, Hornabrook RW, Lambie DG. Comparison of mefenamic acid and propranolol with placebo in migraine prophylaxis. *Acta Neurol Scand* 1986; **73**: 490–492.

119. Tfelt-Hansen P, Standnes B, Kangasneimi P *et al*. Timolol vs propranolol vs placebo in common migraine prophylaxis: a double-blind multicenter trial. *Acta Neurol Scand* 1984; **69**: 1–8.

120. Sudilovsky A, Elkind AH, Ryan RE Sr *et al*. Comparative efficacy of nadolol and propranolol in the management of migraine. *Headache* 1987; **27**: 421–426.

121. Capildeo R, Rose FC. Single-dose pizotifen, 1.5 mg nocte: a new approach in the prophylaxis of migraine. *Headache* 1982; **22**: 272–275.

122. Arthur GP, Hornabrook RW. The treatment of migraine with BC105 (pizotifen): a double-blind trial. *NZ Med J* 1971; **464**: 5–9.

123. Hughes RC, Foster JB. BC105 in the prophylaxis of migraine. *Curr Ther Res* 1971; **13**: 63–68.

124. Lance JW, Anthony M, Somerville B. Comparative trial of serotonin antagonists in the management of migraine. *Br Med J* 1970; **2**: 327–330.

125. Sjaastad O, Stensrud P. Appraisal of BC-105 in migraine prophylaxis. *Acta Neurol Scand* 1969; **45**: 594–600.

126. Graham JR. Headache rounds (pizotifen). The Faulkner Hospital, 26 June 1968.

127. Lance JW, Anthony M. Clinical trial of a new serotonin antagonist, BC-105, in the prevention of migraine. *Med J Aust* 1968; **1**: 54–55.

128. Cleland PG, Barnes D, Elrington SA *et al*. Effectiveness of pizotifen prophylaxis and sumatriptan therapy in migraine. 1st Congress of the European Federation of Neurological Societies, Marseille, France, September 1995 (Poster).

129. Speight TM, Avery GS. Pizotifen (BC-105): a review of its pharmacological properties and its therapeutic efficacy in vascular headaches. *Drugs* 1972; **3**: 159–203.

130. Sorensen PS, Larsen BH, Rasmussen MJK *et al*. Flunarizine versus metoprolol in migraine prophylaxis: a double-blind, randomized parallel group study of efficacy and tolerability. *Headache* 1991; **31**: 650–657.

131. Ziegler DK, Hurwitz A, Preskorn S *et al*. Propranolol and amitriptyline in prophylaxis of migraine. Pharmacokinetic and therapeutic effects. *Arch Neurol* 1993; **50**: 825–830.

132. Ziegler DK, Hurwitz A, Hassanein RS *et al*. Migraine prophylaxis. A comparison of propranolol and amitriptyline. *Arch Neurol* 1987; **44**: 486–489.

133. Couch JR, Hassaneim RS. Amitriptyline in migraine prophylaxis. *Arch Neurol* 1979; **36**: 695–699.

134. Couch JR, Ziegler DK, Hassaneim R. Amitriptyline in the prophylaxis of migraine. Effectiveness and relationship of antimigraine and antidepressant effects. *Neurology* 1976; **26**: 121–127.

135. Klapper J. Divalproex sodium in migraine prophylaxis: a dose-controlled study. *Cephalalgia* 1997; **17**: 103–108.

136. Mathew NT, Saper JR, Silberstein SD *et al*. Migraine prophylaxis with divalproex. *Arch Neurol* 1995; **52**: 281–286.

137. Jensen R, Brinck T, Olesen J. Sodium valproate has a prophylactic effect in migraine without aura: a triple-blind, placebo-controlled crossover study. *Neurology* 1994; **44**: 647–651.

138. Silberstein SD. Divalproex sodium in headache: literature review and clinical guidelines. *Headache* 1996; **36**: 547–555.

139. Murphy JJ, Heptinstall S, Mitchell JRA. Randomised double blind placebo controlled trial of feverfew in migraine prevention. *Lancet* 1988; **ii**: 189–192.

140. Johnson ES, Kadam NP, Hylands DM *et al*. Efficacy of feverfew as prophylactic treatment of migraine. *Br Med J* 1985; **291**: 569–573.

141. Whitmarsh TE, Coleston-Shields DM, Steiner TJ. Double-blind randomized placebo-controlled study of homeopathic prophylaxis of migraine. *Cephalalgia* 1997; **17**: 600–604.

142. Brigo B, Serpelloni G. Homeopathic treatment of migraines: a randomised, double-blind controlled study of sixty cases. *Berlin J Res Homeopathy* 1991; **1**: 98–106.

143. Schoenen J, Lenaerts M, Bastings E. High-dose riboflavin as a prophylactic treatment of migraine: results of an open pilot study. *Cephalalgia* 1994; **14**: 328–329.

144. Schoenen J, Jacquy J, Lenaerts M. Effectiveness of high-dose riboflavin in migraine prophylaxis. A randomized controlled trial. *Neurology* 1998; **50**: 466–470.

145. Mauskop A, Altura BM. Role of magnesium in the pathogenesis and treatment of migraines. *Clin Neurosci* 1998; **5**: 24–27.

146. Peikert A, Wilimzig C, Kohne-Volland R. Prophylaxis of migraine with oral magnesium: results from a prospective, multi-center, placebo-controlled and double-blind randomized study. *Cephalalgia* 1996; **16**: 257–263.

147. Facchinetti F, Sances G, Borella P *et al*. Magnesium prophylaxis of menstrual migraine: effects on intracellular magnesium. *Headache* 1991; **31**: 298–301.

148. Pfaffenrath V, Wessely P, Meyer C *et al*. Magnesium in the prophylaxis of migraine – a double-blind placebo-controlled study. *Cephalalgia* 1996; **16**: 436–440.

149. Melchart D, Linde K, Fischer P *et al*. Acupuncture for idiopathic headache (Cochrane Review). *Cochrane Database Syst Rev* 2001; **1**: CD001218.

150. Farmer K. Biofeedback and headache. In: Cady RK, Fox AW, editors. *Treating the Headache Patient*. New York: Marcel Dekker, 1995; pp. 287–303.

151. Holmes DS, Burish TG. Effectiveness of biofeedback for treating migraine and tension headaches: a review of the evidence. *J Psychosom Res* 1983; **27**: 515–532.

152. Cerbo R, Barbanti P, Fabbrini G *et al*. Amitriptyline is effective in chronic but not in episodic tension-type headache: pathogenetic implications. *Headache* 1998; **38**: 453–457.

153. Dowson AJ. Diagnosis and management of non-migraine headache. *Pharmaceutical J* 2002; **268**: 176–179.

154. Hippisley-Cox J, Pringle M, Hammersley V *et al*. Antidepressants as risk factor for ischaemic heart disease: case-control study in primary care. *Br Med J* 2001; **323**: 666–669.

155. Ekbom K. Treatment of acute cluster headache with sumatriptan. *New Engl J Med* 1991; **325**: 322–326.

156. van Vliet JA, Bahra A, Martin V *et al*. Intranasal sumatriptan is effective in the treatment of acute cluster headache – a double-blind placebo-controlled crossover study. *Cephalalgia* 2001; **21**: 270–271.

157. Bahra A, Gawel MJ, Hardebo J-E *et al*. Oral zolmitriptan is effective in the acute treatment of cluster headache. *Neurology* 2000; **54**: 1832–1839.

158. Kudrow L. Response of cluster headache attacks to oxygen inhalation. *Headache* 1981; **21**: 1–4.

159. Fogan L. Treatment of cluster headache: a double-blind comparison of oxygen versus air inhalation. *Arch Neurol* 1985; **42**: 362–363.

160. Dowson AJ. Analysis of the patients attending a specialist UK headache clinic over a 3-year period. *Headache* 2002; submitted for publication.

161. Dowson AJ. Diagnosis and management of facial pain. *Pharmaceutical J* 2002; **268**: 215–218.

162. Cady RK, Schreiber CP, Billings C *et al*. Subjects with self-described "sinus" headache meet diagnostic criteria for migraine. *Cephalalgia* 2001; **21**: 298 (Abstract).

163. Holmes WF, MacGregor EA, Sawyer JPC *et al*. Information about migraine disability influences physicians' perceptions of illness severity and treatment need. *Headache* 2001; **41**: 343–350.

164. de Lissovoy G, Lazarus SS. The economic cost of migraine. Present state of knowledge. *Neurology* 1994; **44**(Suppl 4): 56–62.

165. Stewart WF, Lipton RB, Kolodner K *et al*. Reliability of the migraine disability assessment score in a population-based sample of headache sufferers. *Cephalalgia* 1999; **19**: 107–114.

166. The Headache Impact Test (HIT). www.amIhealthy.com

167. Dowson AJ. Assessing the impact of migraine. *Curr Med Res Opin* 2001; **17**: 298–309.

168. Kosinski M, Bjorner JB, Dahlof C *et al*. Development of HIT-6, a paper-based short form for measuring headache impact. *Cephalalgia* 2001; **21**: 334 (Abstract).

169. Hackett G, Kerrigan P, Baxendine M *et al*. *Goals of Migraine Management*. Synergy Medical Education, 1994.

170. International Headache Society Clinical Trials Subcommittee. *Guidelines for Controlled Trials of Drugs in Migraine*, 2nd Edition, 2000; www.i-h-s.org

171. Bates D, Ashford E, Dawson R *et al*. Subcutaneous sumatriptan during the migraine aura. *Neurology* 1994; **44**: 1587–1592.

172. Dowson A. Can oral 311C90, a novel 5-HT1D agonist, prevent migraine headache when taken during an aura? *Eur Neurol* 1996; **36**(Suppl 2): 28–31.

173. Sheftell F, O'Quinn S, Watson C *et al*. Low migraine recurrence with naratriptan: clinical parameters related to recurrence. *Headache* 2000; **40**: 103–110.

174. Silberstein S, Mathew N, Saper J *et al*. Botulinum toxin type A as a migraine preventive treatment. *Headache* 2000; **40**: 445–450.

175. Schmitt WJ, Slowey E, Fravi N *et al*. Effect of botulinum toxin A injections in the treatment of chronic tension-type headache: a double-blind, placebo-controlled trial. *Headache* 2001; **41**: 658–664.

176. Porta M. A comparative trial of botulinum toxin type A and methylprednisolone for the treatment of tension-type headache. *Curr Rev Pain* 2000; **4**: 31–35.

177. Rollnik JD, Tanneberger O, Schubert M *et al*. Treatment of tension-type headache with botulinum toxin type A: a double-blind, placebo-controlled study. *Headache* 2000; **40**: 300–305.

178. Saper JR, Winner PK, Lake E III. An open-label dose-titration study of the efficacy and tolerability of tizanidine hydrochloride tablets in the prophylaxis of chronic daily headache. *Headache* 2001; **41**: 357–368.

179. Drake ME, Greathouse NI, Armentbright AD *et al*. Prophylactic treatment of migraine with tizanidine. *Cephalalgia* 2001; **21**: 376 (Abstract).

180. Freitag FG, Diamond S, Diamond ML *et al*. Tizanidine in the preventative treatment of chronic tension type headache. In: *Montreal 2000. Proceedings of the 42nd Annual Scientific Meeting of the American Headache Society, 2000*: p. 208 (Abstract).

181. Smith TR. Low dose tizanidine combined with long-acting NSAIDs for detoxification from analgesic rebound headache, a retrospective review. In: *Montreal 2000. Proceedings of the 42nd Annual Scientific Meeting of the American Headache Society, 2000*: p. 208 (Abstract).

Appendix 1 – Antimigraine Drugs

Acute treatments

Analgesics

Drug (generic name)	Route of administration	Trade name	Formulation	Dose(s)	Side-effects	Comments
Tolfenamic acid	Oral	Clotam Rapid (UK)	Tablet 200 mg	1–2 times per attack	GI upset Skin reactions Dysuria	NSAID Rarely causes reversible liver function changes Licensed in the UK for migraine
Ibuprofen	Oral		Tablet 200, 400, 600, 800 mg	800 mg then q 8 hours PRN	GI upset/ haemorrhage Rash Thrombocytopenia	NSAID Approved in the USA for OTC use
Naproxen	Oral	Naprosyn (UK, USA)	Tablet 250, 375, 500 mg	250–500 mg then q 8 hours PRN	Rash GI intolerance Headache, tinnitus, vertigo Blood, renal, hepatic disorders	NSAID
Ketoprofen	Oral	Ketocid (UK)	Tablet 25, 50, 75 mg	75–100 mg then q 6–8 hours PRN	GI intolerance CNS effects	NSAID
Meclofenamate	Oral		Tablet 100 mg	100 mg then q 8 hours PRN	GI intolerance	NSAID

Combination analgesics

Drug (generic name)	Route of administration	Trade name	Formulation	Dose(s)	Side-effects	Comments
Paracetamol*/ domperidone	Oral	Domperamol (UK)	Tablet 500 mg/10 mg	2–8 tablets per attack	Raised serum prolactin Galactorrhoea Gynaecomastia Reduced libido Rash. Allergic reactions	Analgesic/ antidopaminergic Rarely causes extrapyramidal symptoms Not available in the USA
Isometheptene/ paracetamol*	Oral	Midrid (UK/USA)	Capsule 65 mg/325 mg	2–5 capsules per attack	Dizziness	Sympathomimetic/ analgesic
Isometheptene/ dichloralphenazone/ paracetamol*	Oral	Midrin (USA)	Capsule 65 mg/100 mg/325 mg	2–5 capsules per attack	Dizziness Skin rash	Sympathomimetic/ analgesic Not available in the UK
Aspirin/ metoclopramide	Oral	Migramax (UK)	Powder in sachets 900 mg/10 mg	1–3 sachets per attack	GI upset and haemorrhage Drowsiness Endocrine disorders Extrapyramidal symptoms	Analgesic/ anti-emetic
Paracetamol*/ metoclopramide	Oral	Paramax (UK)	Tablets 500 mg/5 mg	2–6 tablets per attack	Extrapyramidal symptoms Raised serum prolactin Drowsiness. Diarrhoea	Analgesic/ anti-emetic
Paracetamol*/ aspirin/caffeine	Oral	Excedrin (USA)	Tablets 325 mg/326 mg/65 mg	2–8 tablets per attack		OTC analgesic combination Licensed for mild to moderate migraine in the USA Not available in the UK

*Paracetamol is known as acetaminophen in the USA.

Monotherapy and combinations including opiate analgesics

Drug (generic name)	Route of administration	Trade name	Formulation	Dose(s)	Side-effects	Comments
Buclizine/ paracetamol*/ codeine	Oral	Migraleve (UK)	Pink tablets: 6.25 mg/500 mg/8 mg Yellow tablets: 0 mg/ 500 mg/8 mg	2 pink tablets at onset plus up to 6 yellow tablets per attack	Drowsiness	Simple and opiate analgesic/ anti-emetic Not available in the USA
Butalbital/ aspirin/ caffeine/ codeine	Oral	Fiorinol (USA)	50 mg/325 mg/40 mg/ 30 mg		Sedation Risk of rebound and medication overuse	Barbiturate/simple and opiate analgesic Not available in the UK
Butorphanol	Nasal spray	Stadol (USA)	Nasal spray 1 mg	1 spray may be repeated after 1 hour; sequence may be repeated 4 hours after last dose	Dizziness Drowsiness Nausea/vomiting Vertigo Blurred vision Nervousness Taste perversion	Opiate analgesic Primary role in rescue Not available in the UK
Hydromorphone	Suppository		Suppository 3 mg	1–2 suppositories per attack	Constipation Nausea/vomiting Drowsiness Dependence Overuse Impairment of function	Opiate analgesic Primary role in rescue Not licensed for migraine in the UK

*Paracetamol is known as acetaminophen in the USA.

Triptans

Drug (generic name)	Route of administration	Trade name	Formulation	Dose(s)	Side-effects	Comments
Almotriptan	Oral	Almogran (UK) Axert (USA)	Tablet 6.25, 12.5 mg	1–2 tablets (12.5 mg) per attack	Dizziness Somnolence GI upset Fatigue	
Sumatriptan	Oral	Imigran (UK) Imitrex (USA)	Tablet 25, 50, 100 mg	50 or 100 mg (1–3 doses per attack) Maximum 300 mg per attack in the UK and 200 mg in the USA	Pain Heaviness/pressure Fatigue, Dizziness Drowsiness, Weakness Increases in BP	
Sumatriptan	Nasal spray	Imigran (UK) Imitrex (USA)	Nasal spray 5, 20 mg	1–2 doses (20 mg) per attack	Bitter taste Pain Heaviness/pressure Fatigue, Dizziness Drowsiness, Weakness Increases in BP	
Sumatriptan	Subcutaneous injection	Imigran (UK) Imitrex (USA)	Subcutaneous injection 6 mg	1–2 doses (6 mg) per attack, separated by at least 1 hour	Pain at injection site Pain Heaviness/pressure Fatigue, Dizziness Drowsiness, Weakness Increases in BP	

Triptans (continued)

Drug (generic name)	Route of administration	Trade name	Formulation	Dose(s)	Side-effects	Comments
Rizatriptan	Oral	Maxalt (UK, USA)	Tablet 5, 10 mg	1–2 doses (10 mg) per attack in the UK 1–3 doses per 24 hours separated by at least 2 hours in the USA	Dizziness, Somnolence Asthenia, Abdominal/chest pain, Palpitations, Tachycardia GI upset, Musculoskeletal symptoms, CNS disturbances Pharyngeal discomfort Dyspnoea, Pruritus Sweating, Urticaria Blurred vision, Hot flushes Tongue swelling, Rash Toxic epidermal necrolysis Bad taste	
Rizatriptan	Oral	Maxalt Melt	Orally disintegrating tablet 10 mg	1–2 doses (10 mg) per attack in the UK 1–3 doses per 24 hours separated by at least 2 hours in the USA	See above for Maxalt	
Naratriptan	Oral	Naramig (UK) Amerge (USA)	Tablet 1.0, 2.5 mg	1–2 doses (2.5 mg) per attack in the UK 1.0–2.5 mg: may be repeated after 4 hours up to 5 mg per 24 hours in the USA	Malaise, Fatigue, Dizziness Nausea, Pain, Warmth Heaviness or pressure in any part of the body (including the throat and chest) Bradycardia, Tachycardia Visual disturbance	

Triptans (continued)

Drug (generic name)	Route of administration	Trade name	Formulation	Dose(s)	Side-effects	Comments
Eletriptan	Oral	Relpax (UK, USA)	Tablet 20, 40, 80 mg	Unknown at present		Not available yet in the UK and USA
Zolmitriptan	Oral	Zomig (UK, USA)	Tablet 2.5 mg	1–3 doses (2.5 mg) per attack (can increase dose to 5 mg if 2.5 mg is inadequate; maximum 15 mg per attack) in the UK. Doses separated by at least 2 hours and maximum 24-hour dose is 10 mg in the USA	Nausea. Dizziness Warm sensation Asthenia. Dry mouth Somnolence. Heaviness or pressure in throat, neck, limbs or chest. Myalgia Muscle weakness Paraesthesia	
Zolmitriptan	Oral	Zomig Melt	Orally disintegrating tablet 2.5 mg	1–3 doses (2.5 mg) per attack (can increase dose to 5 mg if 2.5 mg is inadequate; maximum 15 mg per attack) in the UK. Doses separated by at least 2 hours and maximum 24-hour dose is 10 mg in the USA	See above for Zomig	

Ergots

Drug (generic name)	Route of administration	Trade name	Formulation	Dose(s)	Side-effects	Comments
Ergotamine/ caffeine	Oral	Cafergot	Tablet 1 mg/100 mg	1–4 tablets per attack (maximum 8 tablets per week)	Nausea, Vomiting Abdominal pain Circulatory impairment Precordial pain Myocardial ischaemia and infarction, Paraesthesia Pleural or retroperitoneal fibrosis	Not available in the UK
Ergotamine/ caffeine	Rectal	Cafergot	Suppository 2 mg/100 mg	1–2 tablets per attack (maximum 4 doses per week)	See above for oral Cafergot	Not available in the UK
Ergotamine/ cyclizine/ caffeine	Oral	Migril (UK)	Tablets 2 mg/50 mg/ 100 mg	1–4 tablets per attack (maximum 6 tablets per week)	See above for oral Cafergot	Available in the UK
Ergotamine	Oral			2 mg	See above for oral Cafergot	Not available in the UK
Ergostine/ caffeine		Ergostat (USA)			See above for oral Cafergot	Not available in the UK
Dihydroergotamine	Subcutaneous injection		Subcutaneous injection 1 mg		Nausea, Vomiting, Dysphoria Flushing, Restlessness Anxiety	Not available in the UK

Ergots (continued)

Drug (generic name)	Route of administration	Trade name	Formulation	Dose(s)	Side-effects	Comments
Dihydroergotamine	Intramuscular injection	DHE 45 Injection	Intramuscular injection		See above for SC injection	Not available in the UK
Dihydroergotamine	Nasal spray	Migranal (USA)	Nasal spray 0.5 mg	4 sprays per attack (2 mg). Maximum 8 sprays per week (4 mg)	Taste alteration. Dizziness Drowsiness Nasal inflammation Nausea. Sore throat, Vomiting Diarrhoea. Dry mouth, Fatigue Hot flushes. Loss of strength Sinus inflammation Stiffness. Tingling	Not available in the UK

Anti-emetics

Drug (generic name)	Route of administration	Trade name	Formulation	Dose(s)	Side-effects	Comments
Prochlorperazine	IM. IV injections			IM/IV 10 mg Suppository 25 mg	CNS disturbances Anticholinergic effects Akathesia ECG and endocrine changes	Phenothiazine Licensed for nausea and vomiting, but used in migraine adjunctively or as a single agent Often used for rescue
Chlorpromazine	IV injection			IV 12.5 mg	CNS disturbances Sedation Akathesia	Phenothiazine Licensed for nausea and vomiting, but used in migraine adjunctively or as a single agent Often used for rescue

Prophylactic treatments

Beta-blockers

Drug (generic name)	Route of administration	Trade name	Formulation	Dose(s)	Side-effects	Comments
Propranolol	Oral	Beta-Prograne (UK) Inderal LA (UK) Syprol (UK)	Sustained release capsule 160 mg Sustained release capsule 160 mg Oral solution 40 mg	20–160 mg daily	Cold extremities CNS and sleep disturbances Bradycardia Exertional tiredness Bronchospasm Heart failure, Hypotension GI upset, Alopecia Thrombocytopenia Dry eyes/skin rash	Non-cardioselective beta-blocker
Metoprolol	Oral	Betaloc (UK) Lopresor (UK)	Tablets 50, 100 mg Tablets 50, 100 mg	50–200 mg daily	See propranolol above	Cardioselective beta-blocker
Timolol	Oral	Betim (UK)	Tablets 10 mg	10–20 mg daily	See propranolol above	Non-cardioselective beta-blocker
Nadolol	Oral	Corgard (UK)	Tablets 40, 80 mg	80–160 mg daily	See propranolol above	Non-cardioselective beta-blocker
Atenolol	Oral		Tablets	25–100 mg daily	See propranolol above	Available in the USA, but not in the UK

5-HT$_2$ antagonists

Drug (generic name)	Route of administration	Trade name	Formulation	Dose(s)	Side-effects	Comments
Methysergide	Oral	Deseril (UK) Sansert (USA)	Tablets 1 or 2 mg	1–3 times daily (UK) 2–8 mg daily (USA)	Inflammatory fibrosis Arterial spasm Nausea, Vomiting, Heartburn Abdominal discomfort Lassitude, Oedema Leg cramps, Dizziness Drowsiness, Weight gain Skin eruptions, Hair loss CNS disturbances	Serotonin antagonist
Cyproheptadine	Oral	Periactin (UK)	Tablets 4 mg	1 every 4–6 hours	Drowsiness Impaired reactions Anticholinergic effects Weight gain	Antihistamine/ serotonin antagonist Not recommended
Pizotifen	Oral	Sanomigran (UK)	Tablets 0.5 or 1.5 mg Elixir 0.25 mg/5 ml	Normally 1.5 mg daily (maximum 4.5 mg daily)	Drowsiness Increased appetite Weight gain	Serotonin antagonist Not available in the USA
Lisuride	Oral			0.075–0.15 mg/day	Sedation Nausea Dizziness	Not available in the UK and USA

Other prophylactic drugs

Drug (generic name)	Route of administration	Trade name	Formulation	Dose(s)	Side-effects	Comments
Clonidine	Oral and transcutaneous patch (USA only)	Dixarit (UK) Clonadine (USA) Catapres patch (USA)	Tablets 25 μg (UK) Tablets/patch 0.1, 0.2, 0.3 mg (USA)	2–3 tablets morning and evening (UK) 1 tablet morning and evening or 1 patch weekly (USA)	Sedation Dry mouth Dizziness Sleeplessness	Central alpha-agonist Not recommended
Divalproex sodium	Oral	Depakote (USA)	Tablets 125, 250, 500 mg	125–1000 mg daily	Liver damage Abdominal pain Abnormal thinking Breathing difficulty Bronchitis, Bruising Constipation, Diarrhoea Dizziness, Emotional changes Fever/flu symptoms Hair loss, Headache Indigestion, Infection Insomnia, Appetite loss Memory loss Nasal inflammation Nausea/vomiting Ringing in the ears Sleepiness, Sore throat Tremor, Vision problems Weakness, Weight gain	Anticonvulsant Licensed for migraine in the USA, but not the UK Teratogenic

Other prophylactic drugs (continued)

Drug (generic name)	Route of administration	Trade name	Formulation	Dose(s)	Side-effects	Comments
Amitriptyline	Oral	Elavil (USA) Lentizol/ Triptafen (UK)	Tablets 10, 25, 50, 75, 100, 150 mg	10–100 mg/day (maximum 200 mg/day)	Anticholinergic effects (e.g. dry mouth) Constipation Urinary retention Vision changes Palpitations and tachycardia Tinnitus Orthostatic hypotension CNS and neuromuscular effects, Gastric irritation Weight changes Allergic skin reactions Jaundice and blood disorders Conduction defects and cardiac arrhythmias Endocrine effects (e.g. changes in libido) Impotence Gynaecomastia and galactorrhoea Changes in blood sugar concentration. Mania or schizophrenic symptoms Withdrawal symptoms	Tricyclic antidepressant Licensed for depression, but not migraine, in the UK Other tricyclic antidepressants used in the USA include: Nortriptyline (10–150 mg/day) Protriptyline (5–30 mg/day)

Other prophylactic drugs (continued)

Drug (generic name)	Route of administration	Trade name	Formulation	Dose(s)	Side-effects	Comments
Fluoxetine	Oral	Prozac (UK/USA)	Capsule	20 mg every other day to 40 mg daily	Insomnia Fatigue Tremor Stomach pain	SSRI Licensed for depression, but not migraine, in the UK
Flunarizine	Oral			5–10 mg/day	Sedation Weight gain, Depression Tremor, Parkinsonism	Calcium channel blocker Not licensed for migraine prevention in the UK and USA
Nimodipine	Oral			120 mg/day	Abdominal discomfort	Calcium channel blocker Not licensed for migraine prevention in the UK
Verapamil	Oral			80–360 mg/day	Constipation	Calcium channel blocker Not licensed for migraine prevention in the UK
Dihydroergotamine				2–3 mg/day	Nausea Headache Dizziness Development of CDH	Ergot alkaloid Not licensed for migraine prevention in the UK and USA

Other prophylactic drugs (continued)

Drug (generic name)	Route of administration	Trade name	Formulation	Dose(s)	Side-effects	Comments
Naproxen	Oral	Naprosyn (UK, USA)		500 mg/day	Dyspepsia GI bleeding Constipation Tinnitus, Bronchospasm	NSAID Not licensed for migraine prevention in the UK
Aspirin	Oral			250 mg/day	See Naproxen above	Not licensed for migraine prevention in the UK
Oestradiol	Percutaneous gel		Percutaneous gel	15 mg/day for 7 days during menstruation	Short-term prevention of migraine associated with menses	

Appendix 2 – Useful Addresses and Websites for the GP and the Patient

For the primary care physician
Societies, journals and congresses

International Headache Society (IHS)
Website: www.i-h-s.org
Journal: *Cephalalgia*
Congress: International Headache Congress (biannual)

American Headache Society (AHS)
Address: 19 Mantua Road, Mt. Royal, NJ 08061, USA
Tel.: (+1) 856 423 0043
Fax: (+1) 856 423 0082
E-mail: ahshq@talley.com
Website: www.ahsnet.org
Journal: *Headache*
Congress: American Headache Society Meeting (annual)

Migraine in Primary Care Advisors (MIPCA)
Address: Maggie Adams (Secretary), Woodstock, Tilford Road, Hindhead, Surrey GU26 6SF, UK
Tel.: (+44) (0)1428 607 837

Primary Care Network
Address: 1230 E. Kingsley Street – Suite G, Springfield, MO 65804, USA
Tel.: (+1) 417 886 2026
Fax: (+1) 417 883 7476
Website: www.primarycarenet.org

British Association for the Study of Headache (BASH)
Address: Carol Taylor (secretariat), Wood Dene, Stanton Lees, nr. Matlock, Derbyshire, DE4 2LQ, UK
Tel.: +44 (0) 1629 733 406
E-mail: carol@caroltaylor.co.uk
Website: www.bash.org.uk

The Migraine Trust
Address: 45 Great Ormond Street, London, WC1N 3HZ, UK
Tel.: +44 (0) 207 831 4818
Fax: +44 (0) 207 831 5174
E-mail: via the website
Website: www.migrainetrust.org
Congress: Migraine Trust International Symposium (biannual)

Websites other than the above containing useful information
Medscape: www.neurology.medscape.com
Doctor's Guide Migraine Site: www.pslgroup.com/migraine.htm
MIDAS website: www.migraine-disability.net
HIT websites: www.amlhealthy.com; www.headachetest.com

For the patient
Societies

World Headache Alliance (WHA)
Address: 612 Thornwood Avenue, Burlington, Ontario, Canada L7N 3B8
E-mail: info@w-h-a.org
Website: www.w-h-a.org

Migraine Trust (see above)

National Headache Foundation (NHF)
Address: 428 W. St. James Place, 2nd Floor, Chicago, IL 60614-2750, USA
Tel.: (+1) 888 643 5552
E-mail: info@headaches.org
Website: www.headaches.org

American Council for Headache Education (ACHE)
Address: 19 Mantua Road, Mount Royal, NJ 08061, USA
Tel.: (+1) 856 423 0258
E-mail: acheq@talley.com
Website: www.achenet.org

Migraine Action Association (UK)
Address: Unit 6, Oakley Hay Lodge Business Park, Great Folds Road, Great Oakley, Northants NN18 9AS, UK
Tel.: +44 (0) 1536 461 333
Fax: +44 (0) 1536 461 444
E-mail: info@migraine.org.uk
Website: www.netdoctor.co.uk

Migraine Association of Canada
Address: 365 Bloor Street East, Suite 1912, Toronto, Ontario, Canada
M4W 3L4
Tel.: (+1) 416 920 4916

Websites other than the above containing useful information
Health Destinations – Headache Site: www.connect2health.com
Primary Care Network – Headache Site: www.headachecare.com
Ronda's Migraine Page Site: www.migrainepage.com
MIDAS website: www.migraine-disability.net
HIT websites: www.amlhealthy.com; www.headachetest.com

Index

*Page numbers followed by 'f' indicate figures; page numbers followed by 't' indicate tables. Main entries are in **bold**.*

This index is in letter-by-letter order whereby spaces and hyphens in main entries are excluded from the alphabetization process.